The EASY EATING DIET Cookbook

150 Fit Food Recipes for Real Life to Get Leaner, Lighter and Healthier

And enjoy delicious and nutritious food without complicated and time-consuming recipes.

SEAN BARKER, CPT, PN2
AUTHOR OF THE AMAZON BEST SELLER, *THE EASY EATING DIET*

The Easy Eating Diet Cookbook
Copyright © 2020 by Sean Barker

All rights reserved. No part of this publication may be reproduced, distributed, or transmitted in any form or by any means, including photocopying, recording, or other electronic or mechanical methods, without the prior written permission of the author, except in the case of brief quotations embodied in critical reviews and certain other non-commercial uses permitted by copyright law.

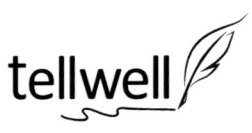

Tellwell Talent
www.tellwell.ca

ISBN
978-0-2288-3989-7 (Hardcover)
978-0-2288-3988-0 (Paperback)
978-0-2288-3990-3 (eBook)

Dedication

This book is inspired by all the passionate home cooks and professional chefs who enjoy sharing healthy, fresh, flavourful food with their family and friends. And for anyone who has ever eaten at our family's table.

DISCLAIMER

All information presented and written within *The Easy Eating Diet Cookbook* and website is intended for informational purposes only. You should not rely on this information as a substitute for medical advice, diagnosis, or treatment. If you have any concerns or questions about your health or diet, you should always consult with a physician, dietician, or other health-care professional. The author and publisher of *The Easy Eating Diet Cookbook* are not doctors, nutritionists, or registered dietitians.

Statements within this book or website have not been evaluated or approved by Health Canada or the Food and Drug Administration. Any products mentioned in this book or website are not intended to diagnose, treat, cure, or prevent any disease. Please consult a doctor before altering your diet in any way or before taking any supplements. You are ultimately responsible for all decisions pertaining to your health and diet. Each individual's dietary needs and restrictions are unique to the individual. The reader assumes full responsibility for consulting a qualified health professional regarding health conditions or concerns and before starting a new diet or health program.

The writers and publishers of this book and website are not responsible for adverse reactions, effects, or consequences resulting from the use of any foods, recipes, or suggestions herein or hereafter. *The Easy Eating Diet Cookbook* occasionally offers nutritional recommendations along with recipes and serving suggestions. This information is provided as a courtesy and is an estimate only. *The Easy Eating Diet Cookbook* and its author and publisher cannot be held responsible for any errors, omissions, or inaccuracies published.

Although *The Easy Eating Diet Cookbook* attempts to provide accurate recipe and serving suggestions, these figures are only estimates. Varying factors such as ingredient product types or brands purchased can change a recipe's result and it's nutritional content. Under no circumstances will *The Easy Eating Diet Cookbook* or its author and publisher be responsible for any loss or damage resulting from your reliance on cooking instructions provided here. By purchasing *The Easy Eating Diet Cookbook* and reading its content, you agree to these terms.

THE EASY EATING DIET COOKBOOK

After the release and positive response of *The Easy Eating Diet* in 2018, the biggest request I had was for more healthy recipes, or an entire *Easy Eating Diet* cookbook. (If you haven't yet, you might also want to read *The Easy Eating Diet* first, as it's filled with twenty-five chapters based on twenty-five years of health and fitness coaching experience, answering many of the most common questions on health, fitness, weight loss, motivation, and mindset. And by not reading it, it would be like watching the sequel to a Marvel movie without watching the first one.) Spoiler alert: *The Easy Eating Diet* isn't really a diet!

So with my passion for fitness and food, I then took on the challenge of writing this second book (at 5 a.m. every morning for over a year), all while I continued operating my fitness business, consulting for other companies, being a husband, and busy dad to a six and twelve-year-old. Oh, and during the outbreak of a worldwide pandemic well-known now as Covid-19, which seemed to, by force of nature, at least get us cooking at home more.

All the cooking, of course, came with lots of messy dishes from experimenting in the kitchen with healthy hacks, new recipes, and twists on our favourite family recipes. (Many thanks to my wife for her help and support in so many ways!) But many recipes came with rave reviews from family and friends, and some with food fails. But, "You can't make an omelette without breaking some eggs," as they say.

Before you dig into the *The Easy Eating Diet Cookbook,* I want you to know two things.

1. I am not a professionally trained chef, just a self-trained fit foodie who has been cooking with enjoyment for over two decades by putting in lots of reps in the kitchen. I realized the importance of learning how to cook at an early age after following my passion for health and fitness. And I quickly learned that seeing as you have to eat, and it's best to eat healthy food most of the time to have a healthy strong body, **you might as well make it look and taste good!**

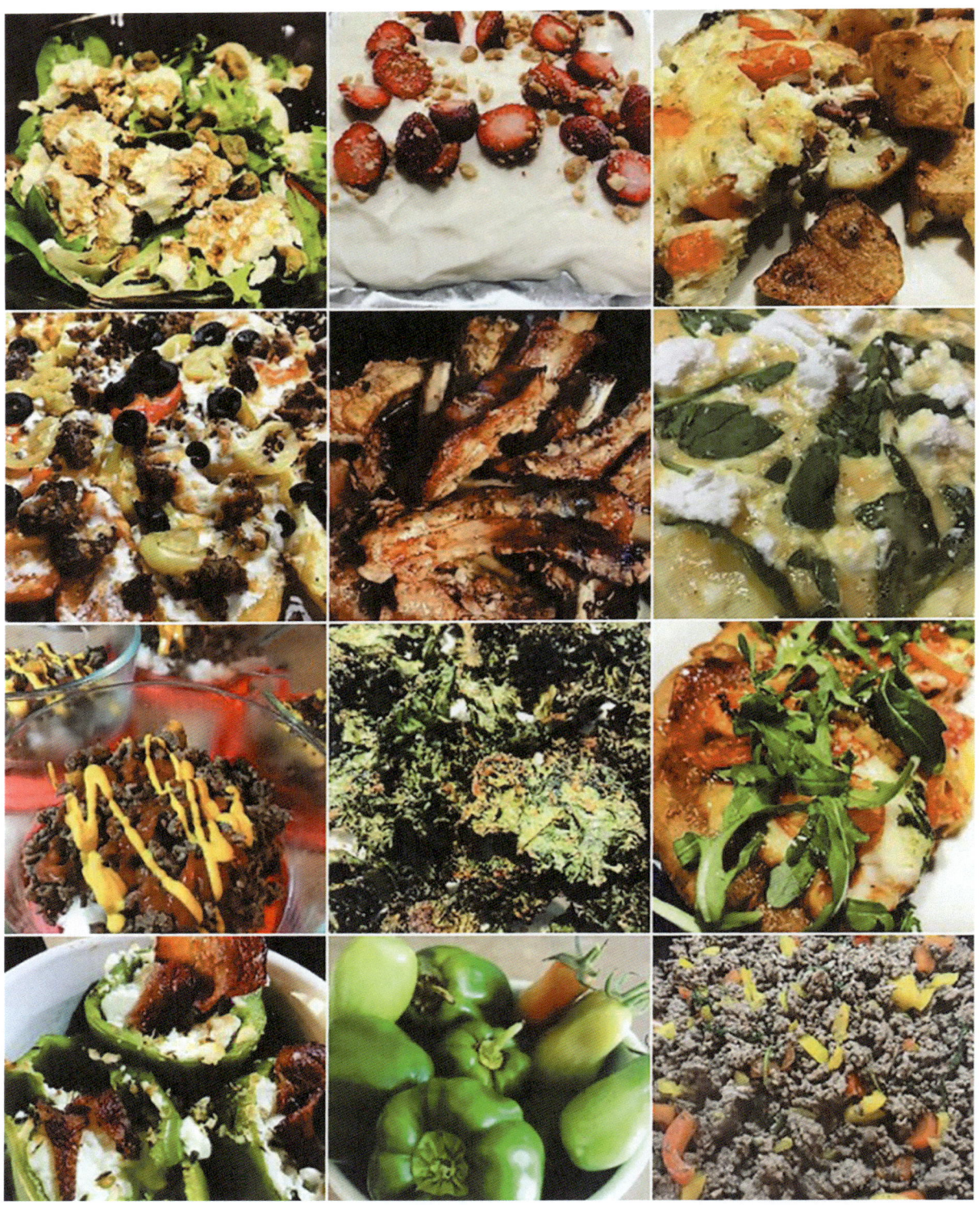

The Easy Eating Diet on Instagram: @sbarker78

2. I don't want you to treat this book like all other cookbooks. I want you to treat cooking like you are a confident chef, (whatever your experience!) by using a **fun and flexible freestyle approach** and not sticking to rigid recipes all the time, with thermometers and teaspoons in hand. Written recipes are included here, of course, and are useful. They give us guidance and confidence in the kitchen. They help us plan, write up shopping lists, and follow methods that serve as a reference point and give us certainty in cooking. Many times, they even inspire us to try some new foods in a new way. But even the best tried and true recipes are just words on paper (or on your screen), until you get into the kitchen, start tasting, and get your hands dirty.

Preparation Time and Tips

I refrained from stating the amount of prep time in each recipe because that can vary greatly depending on the cook, the kitchen tools available, and how busy you are. To feed our family of four, I cook dinner a lot faster on a busy Wednesday night than I do on a slower Saturday night. Some meals will take only minutes to prepare and cook, most just 15-30 minutes, some up to 60 minutes, and very few longer than that, except for using slow cookers and roasting a holiday turkey, of course.

But prep time doesn't always have to be done right before you start cooking.

To save time and food fuss, use one of my *Easy Eating Diet* tips and **"Shop and Chop"** by chopping up a lot of your commonly used fruit and vegetables as soon as you bring them home and *before* you put them away in the fridge. You will also eat more of the healthy stuff and waste less this way! **Pre-portion fresh meats that you buy in bulk** and you will save time and money. Freeze them in plastic zip bags and take them out to thaw so you don't need a chainsaw to get dinner started when you are short on time. Or **pre-cook a big batch of protein like meat, chicken, or fish on a weekend**, to cut normal weekday meal prep time in half.

Servings and Substitutions

Total servings are listed in each recipe but are only approximate recommendations using standard food label guidelines, some testing—depending on how many ingredients you have on hand—and especially whose hands and hunger are at the table. A highly active sixteen-year-old boy just home from hockey practice will need more calories and servings than his forty-five-year-old mother.

With the exception of baking, **most recipes don't need to be treated with perfect precision**, using exact measurements and specific ingredients. Many times (but not always), if you don't have a specific ingredient on hand, similar ingredients that fall under the same category can be used to balance out tastes for sweet, salt, bitter, sour, and umami.

Umami, if unfamiliar to you, is one of the five basic tastes alongside sweet, salty, bitter, and sour. It is Japanese and was discovered over a century ago. It is best described as a savoury or meaty flavour.

You can match your sources of these basic tastes to the style of dish you are preparing. For example, if you need some acidity, it can come from many sources like a crisp cider vinegar, sweet sticky balsamic vinegar, or a squeeze of zesty lemon or lime juice.

You can de-glaze a pan to prevent burning and get all the tasty tidbits clinging to the bottom of the pan, simply with a splash of any wine, broth, stock, or juice you have in your kitchen, or even use plain ole water.

How to Use Herbs and Spices

Especially when it comes to herbs and spices, most of the time, **for fast freestyle weekday cooking for my family, I use ready-to-go dried spices** like garlic powder or an all-in-one bottle of garlic herb or Italian seasoning blend.

Remember, if using fresh herbs, they take a little more time and care and are usually best sprinkled over cooked, finished food, and they also pack a more powerful punch than their dried counterpart cousins, so adjust accordingly. But there is nothing like adding fresh basil over Italian food and fresh cilantro over Mexican food, especially if grown in your own little herb garden! **For herbs and spices, simply add a little if you like a little, and add a little more if you like more.** Dried basil, rosemary, thyme, summer savory, or my favourite go-to, Italian herb, dried oregano, can many times be used interchangeably.

For more of a Mexican smoky spice, a dash of dried cumin, chili powder, or paprika can be swapped. Just be conservative with hotter spices like cayenne and red chili flakes depending on your tolerance and that of others at the table. Even without exotic herbs and spices, the classic dynamic duo of salt and pepper go a long way for simplicity and flavour. I recommend a good, clean sea salt or coarse pink Himalayan or Kosher salt. And for the feisty flavour of freshly ground black pepper, use a pepper grinder for some natural aromatic spice. Can you feel your nose tingling and your mouth salivating already?

Let's awaken your senses, your cooking inspiration, and let your imagination run wild! If you haven't already, **eventually you will learn to add a pinch of salt, to eyeball sprinkles or spoonfuls,** and to taste along the way, for fast freestyle cooking and easy eating. It's how I cook healthy without stress, and it's how I recommend you cook too.

Personal Preferences

Some recipes you may love, some you may like, and some you may not, as that will depend on your personal preference and palate. **Learn the foods and flavours you like** (and of those you are cooking for, of course). Choose a cooking method like grilling, frying, baking, roasting, or toasting. Choose a portion of protein. Surround it with a produce option of colourful vegetables or fruit. Add a small side of starch if you wish, all cooked in, or drizzled with, a little healthy fat or oil and finished with a sprinkle of spice for flavour. Boom! Now you're freestyling. Now you're cooking the easy eating way!

Time and Tenacity

I see too many of the busy parents and professionals I have worked with over the years in my health and fitness coaching business, **stressing out over cooking and eating healthy and complaining about the time it takes.** But then when we do an honest time assessment of their day (something I highly recommend you do if you feel stuck), there is little time put into **weekly meal planning and prep.** More time is spent scrolling through social media or TV at night than actually cooking a healthy meal or prepping for the next day. I hope it's obvious to you which is more important for your health and happiness.

Then I see so many people hopping from one detox or diet trend to another for quick-fix weight loss (where the lost weight always returns). They eventually give up on whipping up simple, delicious, and nutritious food at home for themselves and their families. All because **their diet plan is not sustainable,** or they had a food fail while trying to improve how they eat.

Or worse, those who throw their hands up in the air and too often take the easy way out, but not usually the healthy way out, by choosing to do too many fast food drive-thru dinners after soccer practice with the kids or finger dialling takeout to be delivered to their door.

Social Meals over Media

I prefer you cook and be social at home with family and friends you love, instead of just scrolling through endless recipe blogs, social media clickbait, and "friends" or "followers" you like.

Choose your time more wisely to nourish your body and choose more *implementation over information* **with your diet and lifestyle**, as that is what will actually change your body and your health, for life.

Sure, it's nice to taste with your eyes first and have your food visually appealing, but your food doesn't have to be social media picture perfect. **Freestyle cooking is about simply being a little prepared and relaxing around the kitchen.**

And **for days that you are not prepared, don't stress about it.** Be creative with applying the strategies in this book **and use what ingredients you have on hand**, enjoying the process and being mindful in the moment, from pot to plate.

Cooking simple, wholesome food is one of the most primal and rewarding things you can do. **It's one of the most important life skills to learn and teach your kids.** And if you want to fit into smaller jeans, you've got to embrace your primal genes with good food, fire, and feast!

Like I wrote about in my first book, *The Easy Eating Diet*, **building healthy habits, like exercising or eating better, simply takes a lot of repetition and practice, with a big sprinkle of patience.**

Remember this, **there is no way to fail as long as you keep trying** and look at it like any learning, that you are gaining experience and skills to be better over time.

So, as we all have to eat at least a few times a day for the rest of our lives, I would rather you **look at this cookbook as a guidebook or a meal map to eating easier and healthier**, with many routes to arrive at your destination.

Some recipes are fast and furious, some slow and steady, and some are to just enjoy the ride for pure pleasure. Of course, some are to also help instruct you to eating easier, but more importantly, to **inspire you to be creative and confident in the kitchen,** to cook and eat well for you and others.

The best eating experiences are those you share with family and friends, and "it's just as important who is around your table than what is on it."

"It's just as important who is around your table than what is on it."

Skillpower Over Willpower

Want to know the secret to making eating healthy food easy and eating unhealthy food hard? **It all starts at the grocery store and what you choose to bring home.**

If you bring healthy food home, you, or someone in your household, will eat it. If you bring junk food home, you, or someone in your household, will eat it. That one decision right there is the tipping point that determines if the chips fall in your favour or you end up eating chips.

It's not about having willpower, it's about having skillpower and setting up and controlling your eating environment around you so making better choices are easier, especially at home and even at work.

"It's not about having willpower, it's about having skillpower."

If you spend most of your day away at work, a little meal prepping and packing some healthy food before hand should be accepted and is simply a necessary part of taking care of yourself. **When eating out (aside from special occasions) you shouldn't make it an excuse to overindulge.**

Some of the busiest and most successful people I know, who also travel the most, are also the fittest, so that is not an excuse to not exercise or eat well. I've seen many clients magically drop the unwanted weight and improve their health **simply by packing their own healthy lunch and snacks at home to bring to work or on the road.** You'll also save a lot of money along with saving calories. Having candy within arm's reach at the office also doesn't make eating healthier any easier.

The Food and Feelings System

In all areas of life, **you can't change what you don't acknowledge.** This is especially true of your diet. A great tool for **creating emotional awareness around food** that I use all the time with my clients, is called the ***Food and Feelings System.*** You see, we all have foods that affect us physically and emotionally in different ways, some a little, some a lot. Some foods we should **stop** eating, some we should eat **sometimes**, and others we are **sure** on to eat frequently.

"You can't change what you don't acknowledge."

STOP foods. Stop foods are foods you should stop eating, (except for maybe very rare occasions). Either because they don't help you achieve your goals, you have trouble eating them in reasonable amounts, or they just make you feel bad after the initial and artificial food fix. Often, stop foods are processed foods like chips, candy, cakes, and pastries. Stop foods can also be foods that you're allergic or sensitive to.

SOMETIMES foods. These foods you should simply eat sometimes, and be mindful of, and proceed with caution. Maybe you can eat a little bit without feeling bad, or you can have them as an occasional treat, or you can eat them sensibly at a restaurant with others around but not at home alone. These foods might include things like bread, crackers, pasta, ice cream, granola bars, or seasoned nuts. They're not the worst choices, but they are easy to overeat, high in excess energy, and they're not the most nutritious choice either.

SURE foods. Sure foods should make up most of your diet. You like eating them because they're nutritious with few ingredients and you are sure on how good they make your body and mind feel. You can eat them normally, slowly, and in reasonable amounts because they fill you up to satisfied, not stuffed, and they give you sustained energy. Sure foods are usually real whole foods like fruits and vegetables, lean animal and plant proteins, raw nuts, seeds, and some whole grains.

"Fill up to satisfied, not stuffed"

On your journey to building a better diet and body, create your own ***Stop, Sometimes,*** and ***Sure* foods.** Don't forget calorie-containing drinks too, as that's where many sneaky and sugary calories can weigh you down. Everyone's list will be different.

You might be able to leave cookies in the cupboard untouched for months, whereas another person might turn into a cookie monster knowing they are there.

Or, if you always have a bottle of wine in your house, and especially within arm's reach in your kitchen, you will always find the bottom of the bottle with a couple sips turning into nightly slip-ups and leading to weekly weight gain. Once you have your list, **stock your kitchen with as many Sure foods as possible.** Choose the **Sometimes** foods you allow in your house wisely. And **Stop** foods are to be limited or eliminated entirely. At the very least, **consider reducing the variety of Stop or treat foods in your house**, or keep them for out-and-about special occasions only. Simple nutrition rules, built around your values and goals, can go a long way to prevent emotional overeating and drinking!

You can also look at the **Sure foods as something to consume weekly, Sometimes foods as maybe monthly, and Stop foods as quarterly,** like three to four times a year during main holidays or vacations. Take some pressure off your willpower and rev up your skillpower and **surround yourself with foods that support your short-term and long-term goals.**

And always remember that when you get a flat tire (give in to a food binge) on your journey to better eating, don't then slash your other three tires (by binging even more). Just get back in the driver's seat and get back on track at the very next meal or the next day. **One meal, or day of eating, doesn't make a difference either way,** it's the one after it that determines which direction you go.

"When you get a flat tire on your journey to better eating, don't then slash your other three tires."

EASY EATING ESSENTIALS

Your kitchen doesn't have to look like one from a professional cooking show, but to make cooking and eating easier in this modern world **you obviously need some basic tools and appliances**, like a fridge, an oven, and a stovetop. A microwave, dishwasher, and outdoor BBQ grill, although not absolutely necessary, are common conveniences around most households, and some more modern smaller appliances are just nice to have. And for the days you feel overwhelmed, nothing beats the primal flavour and easy cleanup of simply throwing some meat and veggies on a hot outdoor grill!

Recommended Tools of the Trade

Wooden spoons and spatulas
Chef and prep knives
Small and large non-stick frying pan
Small and large soup pots
Small and large cutting boards
Non-stick baking sheet
Ovenproof casserole dish
Large roasting pan
Parchment paper and aluminum foil
High-powered blender
Mixer and mixing bowls

Food processor
Grater
Mandolin slicer
Strainer/colander
Measuring cups
Measuring spoons
Slow cooker
Rice cooker
Pressure cooker
Air fryer
Sparkling water machine

Quick reference chart

Fahrenheit	Celcius	Gas Mark
250°F	120°C	Gas Mark ½
275°F	135°C	Gas Mark 1
300°F	149°C	Gas Mark 2
325°F	162°C	Gas Mark 3
350°F	176°C	Gas Mark 4
375°F	190°C	Gas Mark 5
400°F	204°C	Gas Mark 6
425°F	218°C	Gas Mark 7
450°F	232°C	Gas Mark 8
475°F	246°C	Gas Mark 9
500°F	260°C	Gas Mark 10

THE HEALTHIEST COOKING OILS

Despite their commonly known name, most of the **vegetable oils** used for commercial and home cooking, and long promoted by large agriculture corporations as "heart healthy," like canola, corn, cottonseed, grapeseed, soybean, sunflower, and safflower oil, among some others, **are not beneficial to your health.** Vegetable oils were non-existent until the early 1900s. But with the invention of certain chemical processes and a need for cheap fat substitutions, the world of fat, and our health, hasn't been the same since.

Vegetables oils are a source of mostly polyunsaturated fats, some monounsaturated, and saturated fats, which are all sources of fats we need in our diet. But it is important to keep in mind that there are two main kinds of polyunsaturated fats: omega-3s and omega-6s. We need to get these two types in a certain balance in order to maintain optimal health. **Most people are simply eating too few omega-3s and way too many omega-6s.** Despite their neutral taste, lower cost, and ability to handle high-temperature cooking, like frying, that is commonly used in restaurants, these highly processed vegetable seed oils contain a very high concentration of omega-6 fatty acids and oxidized chemical compounds contributing to inflammation in the body. These highly unstable fatty acids oxidize and get damaged very easily when exposed to heat, light, or oxygen. Omega-3 essential fatty acids found in foods (like cold water fish, grass-fed beef, avocados, olive oil, and some natural nuts and seeds) have been shown to enhance health, protect against heart disease, and reduce inflammation.

But **commercial vegetable oils are unnaturally produced, highly refined, and extracted using high heat and chemicals.** They can also be partially hydrogenated and contain the proven artery damaging trans fats that are formed when vegetable oils are hardened to make margarine and vegetable shortening.

Thankfully, more and more health-conscious people are becoming aware and less and less people are cooking with these vegetable oils at home these days. However, it's still not enough to just not cook with these oils at home.

Be aware that **most processed foods contain these processed vegetable oils,** so you have to be sure to read labels.

Salad dressings, sauces, condiments, cookies, crackers, and chips are common culprits using canola, soybean, or safflower oil to reduce company costs but improve taste, texture, and keep processed foods shelf stable. So, check your ingredients and **avoid those processed vegetable oils as much as you can** to improve your health, reduce inflammation, and help prevent disease. Choose to cook and consume these healthier natural oils below.

Avocado Oil

This oil, recently made available over the last few years, **is my favourite daily cooking oil**, and is available in bottled oil or even spray. It has one of the highest smoke points, coming in around 520° Fahrenheit, which makes it ideal for really high-heat cooking and grilling or just to use as an all-purpose oil. Avocado oil is rich in monounsaturated fats, specifically, oleic acid or omega-9, so it's considered a heart-healthy oil with the potential to lower LDL "bad" cholesterol.

It has a neutral taste and is also great to apply on your skin for treating skin irritations, such as eczema, psoriasis, cracked heels, dandruff, and insect bites and stings.

Extra-Virgin Olive Oil

High quality extra-virgin olive oil is **probably one of the healthiest oils** you can consume. But it's a little more delicate to heat. The smoke points for olive oils ranges from about 325°F (extra-virgin olive oil) to about 465°F (extra-light olive oil). There's a just-right olive oil for every cooking or baking purpose, due to the varying smoke points and flavour profiles. But mostly choose a high quality 100% extra-virgin cold pressed olive oil in a dark bottle, which prevents rancidity from heat or light. If you grab the cheapest stuff on the shelf, many have been found in testing to be fraudulently diluted with cheap, heavily processed vegetables oils! A quality olive oil should be labeled with a third-party certification, cost a little more, and will also taste like fresh olives with a hint of peppery bitterness. That's the healthy polyphenols and antioxidants. If it tastes sour or smells stinky, it's low quality or has gone bad.

Extra-virgin olive oil is not the best for cooking over medium-high or high heat, but it makes a nice finishing oil on top of dips, salads, soups, or bread or in salad dressings and marinades. Olive oil is resistant to heat damage in low and medium heat applications like slow roasting, baking, and light sautéing, thanks to the stability of the fatty acids and antioxidant capacity of the polyphenols. It also preserves and even enhances the nutrient content and absorption of vegetables when used in cooking.

Olive oil has been around for millennia, and it will continue to stick around and can help you stick around. I happen to love Mediterranean food and the long-living culture, so you'll always find extra-virgin olive oil in my kitchen.

Coconut Oil

This popular and controversial oil is neither a magic panacea nor poison. Having a moderate to low smoke point of 350°F, **it contains 80-90% saturated fat**, which is a higher percentage than butter (about 64% saturated fat), beef fat (40%), and especially olive oil (14%). For years we were told too much saturated fat in the diet is unhealthy because it raises "bad" LDL cholesterol levels, which increases the risk of heart disease. But what's interesting about coconut oil is that it can also give "good" HDL cholesterol a boost. Coconut oil is solid at room temperature so you can use it instead of butter or vegetable shortening to make pie crust and other healthier baked goods that require a solid source of fat. **Coconut oil can bring a mild coconut flavour to your food** so that's important to remember for those who don't like coconut. It's also great as a lotion or natural hair and skin moisturizer, as it has anti-bacterial/anti-fungal properties, and of course it's a must in many Thai dishes, along with coconut milk. I see no problems using **coconut oil in moderation.**

Butter

With its rich, creamy mouthfeel and sublime natural flavour, butter, whether unsalted or salted, is by far **the preferred fat to use for many classic cooking applications**. This includes everything from sauce making to baking, or even just spreading on freshly baked bread. Containing around 60% saturated fat and a moderate smoke point of 350°F, it's **been the go-to grease for years** to enhance the function and flavour of our food. Clarified butter and ghee are the pure, golden butterfat from which the dairy milk solids and water have been removed, allowing it to be heated up to 450°F before it starts to smoke.

Next to avocado oil, **butter is my preferred oil for common cooking, especially eggs.** Remember not to confuse natural butter from a farm (proven over centuries to support healthy cooking), with the industrially made margarine from a factory. Because,"I can't believe they promote that stuff like butter!"

In terms of nutrition and controlling caloric intake, it's important to remember that all cooking oils are still calorie-rich fats. (Fat contains 9 calories per gram, and carbohydrates and protein both contain 4 calories per gram.) Regardless of which oil you are using in your cooking, it's important to pay attention to portion size to avoid overdoing it and to keep calories and fat intake at a reasonable level. A serving size of **oil is generally 1 tablespoon and 120 calories**, so if you are watching your weight, it can add up within your daily calories pretty fast. So be mindful, or measure if you have to, when covering the bottom of your pan or drizzling on top of your food. Using 2-3 tablespoons of oil in a recipe that feeds four people is usually ideal.

GLUTEN GUIDE AND CARB CHEAT SHEET

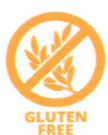
Gluten Free
Almost every recipe is labelled and chosen to be technically **Gluten Free,** which is most important if you have a food sensitivity to gluten-containing foods (like me) and especially important if you have celiac disease (an auto-immune condition where you have to avoid gluten 100%). Most of the recipes are naturally gluten free but please use your own discretion in using certain ingredients as cross contamination in foods, processing, and preparation can occur.

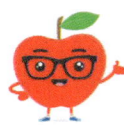
Smart Carb
Some recipes are labelled as **Smart Carb,** meaning they contain some starchy carbohydrates (approximately 20-30 grams of carbs per serving) but are also high in fibre, which helps reduce blood sugar spikes from excess carb intake and is important for intestinal health and regularity. Some examples are oats, beans, legumes, fruit, and starchy vegetables like potatoes and squash.

Low Carb
Most of the recipes are labelled as **Low Carb.** This symbol means it contains low carbohydrates (approximately 15-20 grams of carbs per serving), helping to control blood sugar and high energy calories.

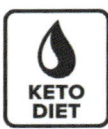
Keto
Many recipes are labelled as **Keto** (short for ketogenic diet). This means it contains very low if any carbohydrates at all per serving (approximately less than 5-10 grams of carbs per serving). But more high-fat ingredients are added to provide energy, taste, and texture. And yes, calories still count in weight loss, whether they are from carbs or fats, and whether you count them or not, **energy balance still counts.**

Other dietary restrictions and food preferences are not directly listed under each recipe, like Dairy Free, Vegan, Vegetarian, Paleo, Low FODMAP etc., but **easy eating substitutions can be made in most recipes**. Choose common alternatives if you desire, like nut flours, dairy-free nut milks, and/or vegan cheese, and vegan plant-based protein sources like beans, legumes, nuts, seeds, tofu, quinoa, and plant protein powder.

A **low FODMAP diet has personally benefited me, and many of my clients, by improving digestion issues** from many so-called healthy foods. (FODMAP stands for Fermentable Oligosaccharides, Disaccharides, Monosaccharides, and Polyols.) These are short chain carbohydrates and sugar alcohols that are poorly absorbed by the body for some people with irritable bowel syndrome (IBS) or similar gut health digestive issues, resulting in abdominal pain, gas, and bloating when eating many commonly known "healthy" foods.

The list of high and low FODMAPS foods are quite extensive and can be found with a simple Google search, but if you are dealing with any uncomfortable digestion issues, omitting some of the most common high FODMAP foods in some recipes, like onions, garlic, beans, and sugar alcohols commonly found in protein bars, can help you reduce bloating, gas and discomfort.

And by **choosing low FODMAP, low-gas causing fruits and vegetables** you can still get a wide variety of micro-nutrients and maintain great health, with foods like blueberries, strawberries, oranges, pineapple, cantaloupe, spinach, bell peppers, green beans, cucumbers, carrots, zucchini, potatoes, squash, and white rice.

The best diet is always the one YOU will follow consistently and that makes YOU feel your best, so simply choose nutritious foods that you like, that like you, and that provide you with high-quality protein, some carbs and fats.

"The best diet is always the one you will follow consistently and that makes you feel your best"

TABLE OF CONTENTS

Disclaimer v
The Easy Eating Diet Cookbook 1
Easy Eating Essentials 10
The Healthiest Cooking Oils 12
Gluten Guide and Carb Cheat Sheet 16
Breakfast 21
Lunch or Dinner 43
Seafood 85
Pizza 95
Snacks, Sides and Sauces 107
Soups and Salads 123
Sweet Treats 135
50 Easy Eating Super Smoothies 155
Thank You 175

BREAKFAST

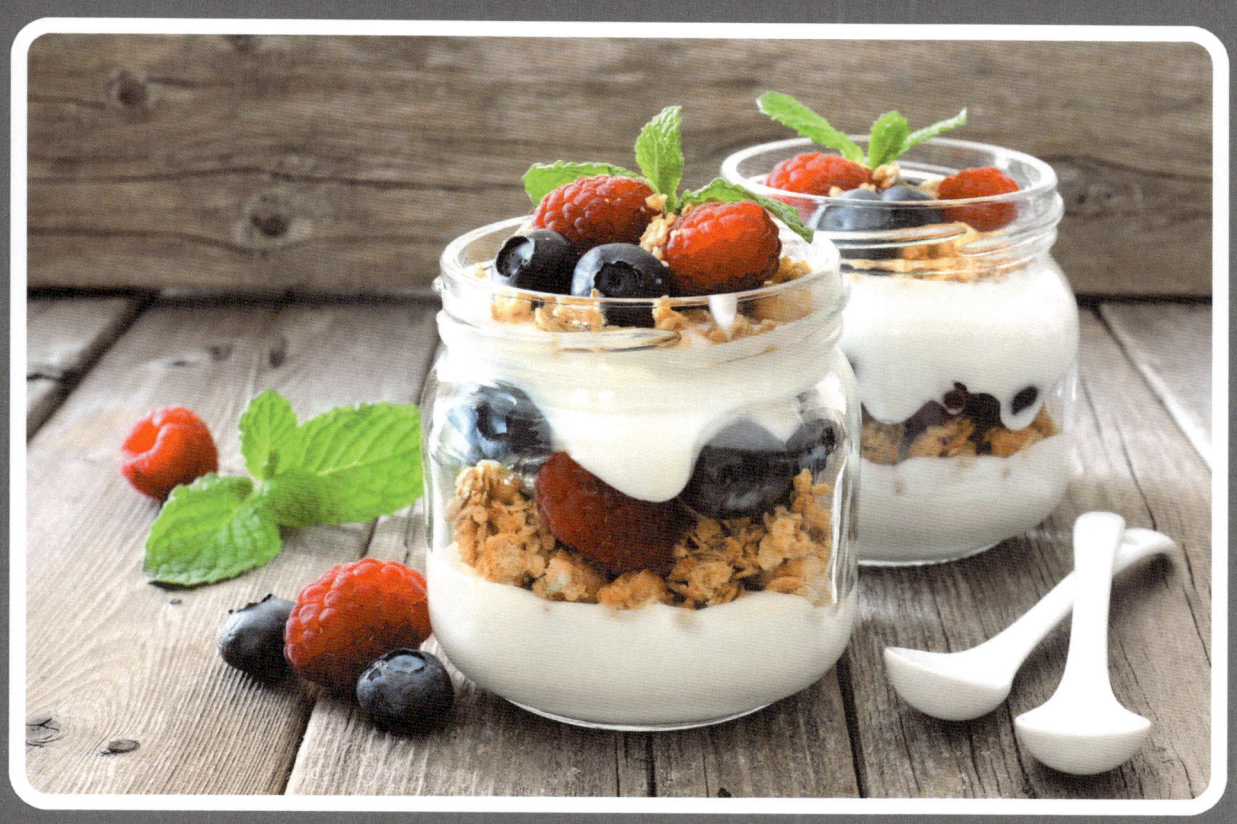

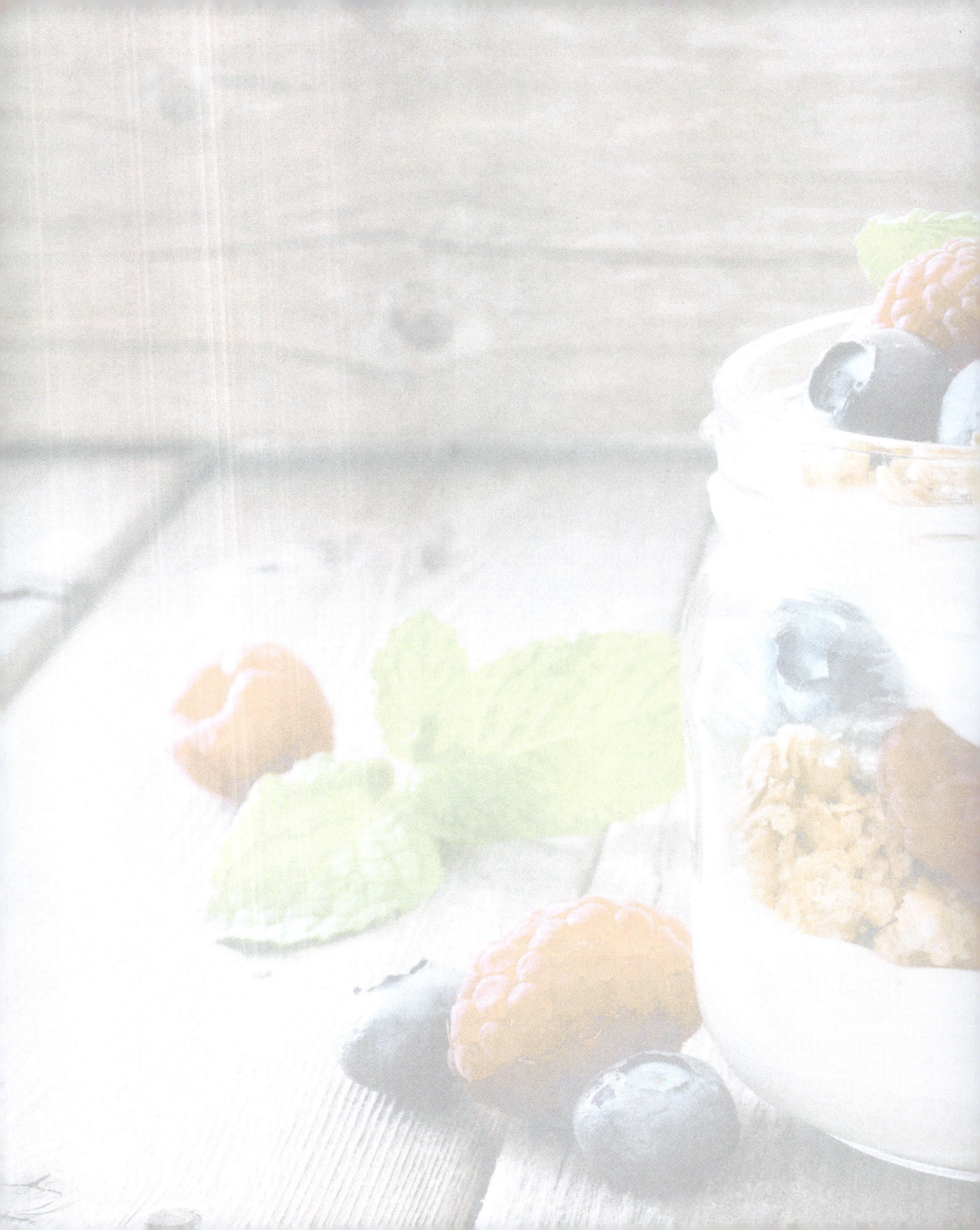

VANILLA CINNAMON PRO-OATS (PROTEIN OATMEAL)

Start the day like a PRO! The answer to a nutritious and delicious breakfast in under two minutes is what I call ProOATS.

Ingredients

1/2 cup of old fashion oats (choose gluten free if preferred)
1/2 cup of water or milk (any kind), or as much as needed for preferred texture

1 scoop of vanilla whey or plant protein powder
1/3 cup of blueberries
Pinch of sea salt
1 tsp of cinnamon

Instructions

Place dry oats in a bowl. Add water or milk, and salt. Microwave for 1 minute. Remove, stir, and let cool for 30 seconds. Add vanilla protein powder. Stir to combine. Add blueberries and cinnamon. Stir one more time and enjoy!

1 serving.

Other ProOATS topping ideas: raspberries, strawberries, hemp hearts, ground flaxseeds, chia seeds, or crushed nuts.

Gluten Free. Smart Carb.

CHOCOLATE NUT BUTTER PRO-OATS (PROTEIN OATMEAL)

Ingredients

1/2 cup of old fashion oats (choose gluten free if preferred)

1/2 cup of water or milk (any kind), or as much as needed for preferred texture

1 scoop of chocolate whey or plant protein powder

1 Tbsp of natural peanut butter or almond butter

Pinch of sea salt

Instructions

Place dry oats in a bowl. Add water or milk, and salt. Microwave for 1 minute. Remove and let cool for 30 seconds. Add chocolate protein powder. Stir to combine. Add peanut butter or almond butter. Stir one more time and enjoy!

1 serving.

Other ProOATS topping ideas: raspberries, strawberries, hemp hearts, ground flaxseeds, chia seeds, or crushed nuts

Gluten Free. Smart Carb.

PEANUT BUTTER BERRY OVERNIGHT OATS

Do you want two extra minutes of sleep in the morning and no time for 1-minute ProOATS? Then get ahead of the game the night before, with Overnight Oats!

Ingredients

1/2 cup of old fashion oats (choose gluten free if preferred)
1 Tbsp chia seeds
1/2 scoop of vanilla whey or plant protein powder
1/2 tsp of cinnamon
1 Tbsp of peanut butter or almond butter

1/2 cup milk (any kind)
1/2 cup berries (fresh or frozen blueberries, raspberries, or sliced strawberries)
Drizzle of maple syrup or honey, if desired

Instructions

In an 8 oz glass mason jar or similar size container combine the oats, cinnamon, chia seeds, protein powder, and nut butter. Add a splash of the milk and mix the nut butter into the oats. Then add the rest of the milk and stir to combine. Top with your fruit of choice or wait to top the oats until you are ready to serve. Place the lid on the jar and refrigerate overnight, or up to 5 days. When you're ready to serve, add a drizzle of maple syrup or honey, if you'd like, and enjoy chilled. Use a larger 16 oz mason jar or larger container if you want more room for larger servings.

1 serving.

Gluten Free. Smart Carb.

BANANA BREAD OVERNIGHT OATS

Ingredients

1/2 cup of old fashion oats (choose gluten free if preferred)
1/2 mashed ripe banana
1/2 cup milk (any kind)
1/2 scoop of vanilla whey or plant protein powder
1 Tbsp of chopped pecans or walnuts
1 tsp vanilla extract
1/2 tsp cinnamon
Drizzle of maple syrup or honey, if desired

Instructions

In an 8 oz glass mason jar, or similar size container, combine the oats, cinnamon, and protein powder. Add a splash of the milk and mix the mashed banana into the oats, or wait to top the oats with sliced banana until you are ready to serve. Then add the rest of the milk and stir to combine. Place the lid on the jar and refrigerate overnight, or up to five days. When you are ready to serve, add a drizzle of maple syrup or honey, if you'd like, and enjoy chilled. Use a larger 16 oz mason jar or larger container if you want more room for larger servings.

1 serving.

Gluten Free. Smart Carb.

BAKED BERRY OATMEAL

Is this oatmeal? Is it squares? Or cookies? This Baked Berry Oatmeal has the taste and texture of all three, so the little extra time it takes to prepare is "berry" well worth it!

Ingredients

3/4 cup walnuts, roughly chopped
2 cups old fashion oats (choose gluten free if preferred)
1 tsp baking powder
1 tsp cinnamon
1/2 tsp nutmeg
1/2 tsp salt

1 3/4 cup milk (any kind)
1/3 cup maple syrup
2 large eggs
3 Tbsp unsalted butter or melted coconut oil
2 cups mixed berries, fresh or frozen
Plain Greek yogurt (optional)

Instructions

Preheat the oven to 375°F. Spray a 9x9 inch baking pan with cooking spray, or line with parchment paper. Start by toasting the walnuts in a pan until fragrant, about 4-5 minutes. Remove walnuts from pan and roughly chop; set aside. In a medium bowl, mix together oats, walnuts, cinnamon, nutmeg, baking powder, and salt. In a small bowl, whisk together milk, maple syrup, eggs, butter, and vanilla. Pour wet mixture into the bowl with the oats. Stir in mixed berries then spread mixture evenly in baking dish. Bake for 40-45 minutes or until golden brown on top. Serve with a dollop of Greek yogurt if you wish.

6 servings.

Gluten Free. Smart Carb.

BLENDER BANANA BERRY PROTEIN PANCAKES

Ditch the pancake powder in a box and go with this nutritious and delicious way to serve up pancakes for the family for a weekend breakfast or even weekday lunch leftovers for picky eating kids. They will flip out for it!

Ingredients

- 2 cups of old fashion oats (choose gluten free if preferred)
- 1 1/4 cups milk (any kind)
- 1 ripe banana
- 1/2 cup of blueberries or dark chocolate chips
- 1 scoop of vanilla whey or plant protein powder
- 1/2 tsp cinnamon
- 1 Tbsp honey
- 1/4 tsp sea salt
- 1 tsp pure vanilla extract
- 1 1/2 tsp baking powder
- 1 egg
- Avocado oil, coconut oil, or butter for cooking

Instructions

Place all ingredients, except egg, blueberries, and cooking oil in the base of a blender and blend until smooth. Add egg and pulse a few times until egg is fully incorporated. Heat a griddle or large sauté pan over medium heat and melt a teaspoon or two of cooking oil. When hot, pour or scoop the batter onto the griddle, using approximately 1/4 cup for each pancake. Top each pancake with 1 Tbsp of blueberries or dark chocolate chips. Watch for bubbles forming on exposed side (about 2-3 minutes). Flip pancake and brown second side for 2-3 minutes more. Remove from pan and serve hot with a drizzle of maple syrup. *If batter becomes too thick to pour easily, add a tablespoon or two of milk to thin.

Makes 8-10 palm-size pancakes.

Gluten Free. Smart Carb.

BLENDER CHOCOLATE PEANUT BUTTER PROTEIN PANCAKES

Dig into these decadent dessert-like pancakes topped with lip-smacking peanut butter, and breakfast will be the most important meal of your day.

Ingredients

2 cups of old fashion oats (choose gluten free if preferred)
1 1/4 cups milk (any kind)
1 ripe banana
1 scoop of chocolate whey or plant protein powder
1 Tbsp of melted peanut butter
1/2 tsp cinnamon

1 Tbsp honey
1/4 tsp sea salt
1 tsp pure vanilla extract
1 1/2 tsp baking powder
1 egg
Avocado oil, coconut oil, or butter for cooking

Instructions

Place all ingredients, except egg and cooking oil, in the base of a blender and blend until smooth. Add egg and pulse a few times until egg is fully incorporated. Heat a griddle or large sauté pan over medium heat and melt a teaspoon or two of cooking oil. When hot, pour or scoop the batter onto the griddle, using approximately 1/4 cup for each pancake. Watch for bubbles forming on exposed side (about 2-3 minutes). Flip pancake and brown second side for 2-3 minutes more. Remove from pan and and serve hot with a drizzle of maple syrup or melted peanut butter.

*If batter becomes too thick to pour easily, add a tablespoon or two of milk to thin.

Makes 8-10 palm-size pancakes.

Gluten Free. Smart Carb.

LOW CARB CREAM CHEESE PANCAKES

You can have your pancakes and eat them too! With these low carb cream cheese pancakes that blend up and cook up fast for an easy eating breakfast.

Ingredients

1/2 cup almond flour
1/2 cup full fat cream cheese
4 eggs
1 tsp granulated natural sweetener
1/2 tsp baking powder
1/2 tsp cinnamon
Avocado oil, coconut oil, or butter for cooking

Instructions

Mix all ingredients in a blender. Fry pancakes in melted oil in a non-stick pan or griddle over a medium heat. If you heat the pan too much, these low carb pancakes will burn easily. I recommend keeping the pancakes on the small side (around palm size), as almond flour pancakes are thinner and more fragile than regular pancakes because of the lack of gluten.

Makes 8-10 palm-size pancakes.

Gluten Free. Low Carb. Keto

GREEK YOGURT AND BERRIES

A "berry" quick and easy protein packed breakfast or snack in under a minute.

Ingredients

1 cup of plain Greek yogurt
1/2 cup of berries
1 Tbsp of chopped pecans, slivered almonds, or crushed walnuts

1/2 tsp of cinnamon
Drizzle of maple syrup or honey, if desired

Instructions

Place yogurt in a bowl. Add berries, nuts, cinnamon, and maple syrup or honey, if desired.

1 serving.

Gluten Free. Smart Carb.

ITALIAN GOAT CHEESE OMELETTE

Omelettes are an "eggcellent" way to get a high protein and produce breakfast, or even an easy eating dinner, in just 5 minutes "flat."

Ingredients

2 Tbsp unsalted butter or avocado oil
1/2 tsp salt
1 tsp black pepper
3 whole eggs, whisked

1/2 cup baby spinach, chopped
2 oz crumbled goat cheese
1 Tbsp of basil pesto

Instructions

Heat butter or oil in a non-stick pan over medium heat. In a small mixing bowl, whisk eggs until frothy. Sprinkle salt and pepper into eggs and whisk again to evenly combine the egg and seasonings. Pour eggs into pan and allow to cook until almost set. Place spinach, goat cheese, and basil pesto over half of the omelette, and fold the opposite side over top of the filling using a spatula. Remove from heat, and carefully slide the omelette onto your plate, using the spatula to loosen any egg that is stuck to the pan. *Use a good store-bought basil pesto with olive oil or use our homemade pesto recipe in this book.

1 serving.

Gluten Free. Low Carb. Keto.

TEXAN TACO OMELETTE

Ingredients

2 Tbsp unsalted butter or avocado oil
1/2 tsp salt
1 tsp black pepper
3 whole eggs, whisked

1/2 cup of cooked ground beef
2 oz shredded Tex-Mex cheese blend
1/4 cup chopped bell or hot banana peppers

Instructions

Heat butter or oil in a non-stick pan over medium heat. In a small mixing bowl, whisk eggs until frothy. Sprinkle salt and pepper into eggs and whisk again to evenly combine the egg and seasonings. Pour eggs into pan and allow to cook until almost set. Place cooked ground beef, Tex-Mex cheese and peppers over half of the omelette, and fold the opposite side over top of the filling using a spatula. Remove from heat, and carefully slide the omelette onto your plate using the spatula to loosen any egg that is stuck to the pan.

1 serving.

Gluten Free. Low Carb. Keto.

MEXICAN CHOPPED CHICKEN OMELETTE

Ingredients

2 Tbsp unsalted butter or avocado oil
1/2 tsp salt
1 tsp black pepper
3 whole eggs, whisked
1/2 cup of cooked chopped chicken breast
2 oz shredded cheddar cheese
1/4 cup chopped bell or hot banana peppers
1 Tbsp of salsa
1 Tbsp of sour cream
1 Tbsp of guacamole

Instructions

Heat butter or oil in a non-stick pan over medium heat. In a small mixing bowl, whisk eggs until frothy. Sprinkle salt and pepper into eggs, and whisk again to evenly combine the egg and seasonings. Pour eggs into pan and allow to cook until almost set. Place cooked chopped chicken, cheddar cheese, and peppers over half of the omelette, and fold the opposite side over top of the filling using a spatula. Remove from heat, and carefully slide the omelette onto your plate, using the spatula to loosen any egg that is stuck to the pan. Top with salsa, sour cream, and guacamole.

1 serving.

Gluten Free. Low Carb. Keto.

DENVER DINER OMELETTE

Ingredients

2 Tbsp unsalted butter or avocado oil
1/2 tsp salt
1 tsp black pepper
3 whole eggs, whisked

1/4 cup of finely chopped ham
1/4 cup of finely chopped bell pepper
1/4 cup of finely chopped onion
2 oz shredded mozzarella cheese

Instructions

Heat 1 Tbsp of butter or oil in a non-stick pan over medium heat. Toss ham, bell pepper, and onion in pan and cook for 5-7 minutes, stirring often until brown and soft. In a small mixing bowl, whisk eggs until frothy. Sprinkle salt and pepper into eggs, and whisk again to evenly combine the egg and seasonings. Heat remaining 1 Tbsp of butter or oil in pan. Pour egg mixture over ham and vegetables, then sprinkle cheese over. Cook until eggs set, and fold the opposite side over top of the filling using a spatula. Remove from heat, and carefully slide the omelette onto your plate, using the spatula to loosen any egg that is stuck to the pan.

1 serving.

Gluten Free. Low Carb. Keto.

OMELETTE MINI MUFFINS

Omelette mini muffins are perfect for easy weekend meal prep. They also make for a fast weekday breakfast or mid-day snack, are high in protein and vegetables, and are a lot healthier than grabbing a regular muffin at the coffee shop.

Ingredients

1/2 cup sun-dried tomatoes, sliced
1 cup baby spinach, finely diced
1/2 onion, finely diced
4 large basil leaves, finely diced

Salt and pepper, to taste
8 large eggs
1/4 cup milk (any kind)
1/3 cup feta cheese crumbles

Instructions

Preheat oven to 350ºF and spray a 12-cup, non-stick muffin tin with cooking spray or use non-stick liners. Finely dice sun-dried tomatoes, spinach, basil, and yellow onion. Then spread out veggies among the 12 cups. Add about 1 teaspoon of feta cheese crumbles to each cup. In a medium bowl, whisk together eggs and milk. Pour egg mixture evenly on top of veggies to fill each cup around 3/4 full. Use a fork or knife to mix, making sure the veggies are evenly distributed within the egg. Season the top of each egg cup with salt and pepper to taste, and then bake at 350ºF for around 18-20 minutes.

Yields 12 mini muffins.

Gluten Free. Low Carb. Keto.

SOFT AND SIMPLE SCRAMBLED EGGS

Almost anyone can simply scramble eggs, but very few can master this delicate dish that only takes minutes. Here's how to crack the code on whipping up a moist and fluffy pan of nature's perfect protein.

Ingredients

2 Tbsp unsalted butter or avocado oil
3 eggs
1/2 tsp salt

1 tsp black pepper
1 Tbsp of whole milk

Instructions

Melt the butter or oil in a medium non-stick pan over medium-low heat. Crack eggs into a bowl, add milk, salt, and pepper and whisk vigorously with a whisk or fork until well blended and you see tiny air bubbles. When the butter begins to bubble, pour in the eggs and immediately use a silicone spatula to gently swirl in small circles around the pan, without stopping, until the eggs look slightly thickened and very small curds begin to form, about 30 seconds. Change from making circles to making long sweeps across the pan until you see larger, creamy curds, about 20 seconds. When the eggs are softly set and slightly runny in places, remove the pan from the heat and leave for a few seconds as they will continue cooking. Give eggs a final stir and serve immediately. Serve with a few fresh chopped chives, if desired.

1 serving.

Gluten Free. Low Carb. Keto.

Eggcellent Eggs Tips:

- Whisk the eggs fast and furious in a bowl, producing air for fluffier eggs.
- Use a good non-stick pan (even keeping one pan just for cooking eggs).
- Butter is best for cooking, but avocado oil works well too, as it has neutral taste.
- Use a soft silicone spatula to swirl and sweep the scrambled eggs.
- Use low and slow heat to prevent bland and browned scrambled eggs.
- Account for carry-over cooking, so remove the pan from the heat a little early.

SOUTHWEST SCRAMBLE

When you want to mix things up with your breakfast, and also cook for your partner, you can simply change direction with this Southwest Scramble.

Ingredients

6 Eggs
2 Tbsp milk
2 Tbsp butter or avocado oil
1 lb loose ground pork sausage
1/2 cup chopped onion
1/2 cup chopped red bell pepper

2 cups chopped, cooked potatoes
Salt and pepper, to taste
1/4 tsp paprika
1/2 tsp garlic powder
1 cup shredded cheese

Instructions

Whisk eggs in a small bowl. Add milk and set aside. Melt 1 Tbsp of butter or oil in large non-stick skillet. Add ground sausage, breaking it up as it cooks. Cook for about 10 minutes over medium-high heat, or until cooked through. Move cooked ground sausage to a plate. Add remaining Tbsp of butter or oil to skillet if needed. Add onion, pepper, cooked potatoes, and spices. (For fast cooked potatoes, poke 2 potatoes with a fork, wrap potatoes in paper towel, and microwave for 10 minutes and let cool). Cook vegetables for 5-10 minutes or until they are cooked through and potatoes are slightly brown. Pour egg mixture over veggies and cook on medium-low heat for 3-5 minutes, stirring and scrambling ingredients in pan until eggs are almost cooked through. Add ground sausage back into skillet, stir to combine, and top with cheese.

2 servings.

Gluten Free. Smart Carb.

FIT BODY FRITTATA

Even though the word Frittata in Italian means fried, a frittata is a fancy Italian way to serve up a baked omelette for brunch, lunch, or even dinner.

Ingredients

8 eggs
1/3 cup heavy whipping cream
3/4 cup shredded mozzarella, cheddar, or goat cheese
Salt and pepper, to taste
Pinch of red pepper flakes

2 Tbsp. avocado oil
1/4 cup chopped mushrooms
1/4 cup chopped bell pepper
1/4 cup sun dried tomatoes
2 cups baby spinach, chopped

Instructions

Preheat oven to 375°F. In a medium bowl, whisk together eggs and heavy cream. Add cheese and vegetables and whisk again. Season with salt, pepper, and a pinch of red pepper flakes. Pour egg mixture into a 9-inch square or round baking dish, greased with avocado oil. Bake for 30-40 minutes or until eggs are set and slightly brown.

4 servings.

Gluten Free. Low Carb. Keto.

BRUNCH STUFFED PORTOBELLO MUSHROOMS

Impress any overnight house guests "rooming" with you, by serving up these fancy and flavourful mush-rooms the next morning, for breakfast or brunch.

Ingredients

1 Tbsp extra-virgin olive oil
2 cloves garlic, minced
1 cup cherry tomatoes, halved
4 cups baby spinach
Salt and pepper, to taste
Pinch red pepper flakes

4 portobello mushrooms, stems removed
4 large eggs
1 cup shredded mozzarella cheese
Freshly chopped parsley

Instructions

Preheat oven to 375°F. Heat oil in a large skillet over medium heat. Add garlic and cook until fragrant, approximately 1 minute. Add cherry tomatoes and cook until starting to burst, usually 5 minutes. Add spinach and cook for 2 minutes more, until wilted. Season with salt, pepper, and a pinch of red pepper flakes. Place mushrooms stem side up on a small baking sheet. Spoon spinach mixture into each mushroom. Crack eggs over spinach and sprinkle cheese over egg. Bake until whites are just set, about 30 minutes. Garnish with parsley before serving.

4 servings.

Gluten Free. Low Carb. Keto.

SAUSAGE STUFFED PEPPERS WITH EGG AND GOAT CHEESE

A gourmet-looking and tasty meal that comes together in minutes, to stuff yourself for breakfast or brunch.

Ingredients

1 Tbsp extra-virgin olive oil
1 Tbsp of butter
1 lb of ground Italian or pork sausage
4 bell peppers, top and stems removed
4 eggs
4 Tbsp of crumbled goat cheese
Salt and pepper, to taste
Freshly chopped parsley, chopped

Instructions

Add 1 Tbsp of olive oil to frying pan. Add ground sausage, breaking it up as it cooks. Cook for about 10 minutes over medium-high heat, or until cooked through. Move cooked ground sausage to a bowl. Fill a microwave-safe glass dish or deep plate with about 1 inch of water. Stand the bell peppers up in the glass baking dish with the open side of the pepper facing down so they steam from the inside. Cook your bell peppers in the microwave on the high setting between 4 to 6 minutes to soften the peppers. Remove peppers from microwave to let cool (plate will be hot so be careful!). While waiting for them to cool, heat a large non-stick skillet with butter and fry 4 eggs, sprinkled with salt and pepper, sunny side up. Stuff each upright open pepper 3/4 full with cooked sausage, then 1 fried egg and top with a little crumbled goat cheese and freshly chopped parsley.

4 servings.

Gluten Free. Low Carb. Keto.

LUNCH OR DINNER

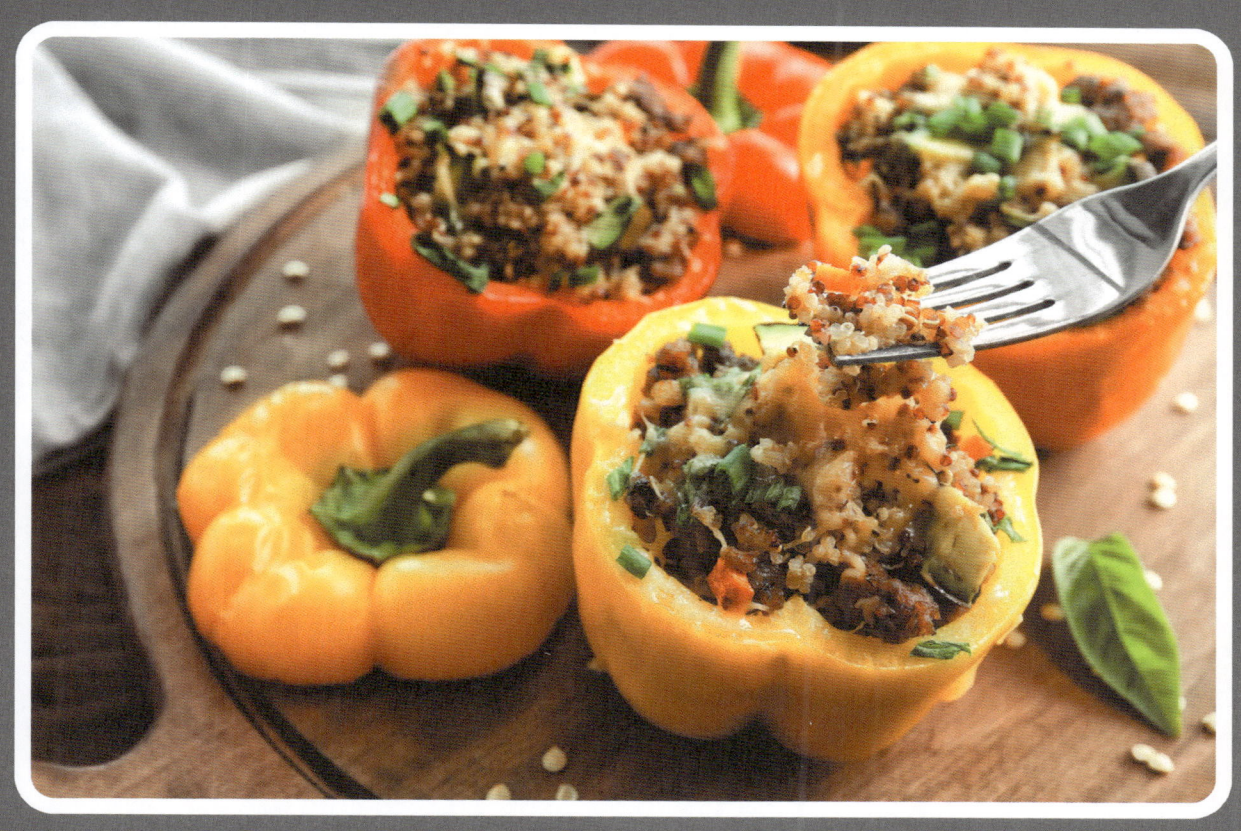

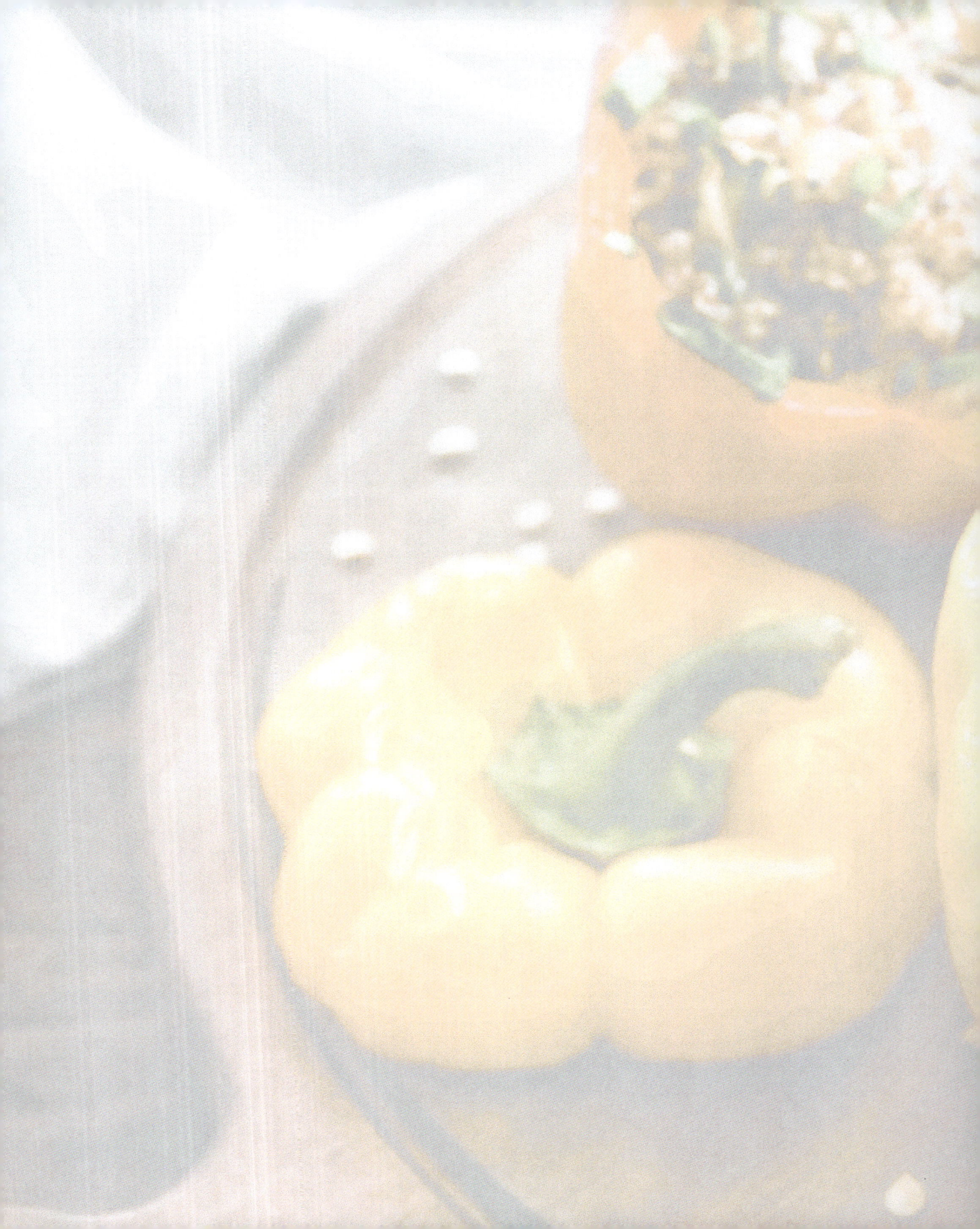

EASY EGG ROLL BOWL

Wrap up a delicious dinner without the wrapper, in just 20 minutes with this one-pan, Asian inspired, Easy Egg Roll Bowl.

Ingredients

1 lb ground beef, chicken, turkey, or pork
2 Tbsp sesame oil, divided
2 garlic cloves, minced
3 green onions, minced
16 oz or 450g coleslaw mix (it will cook down)
2 Tbsp soy sauce (gluten free if preferred)
1/2 tsp sriracha sauce (more for garnish)
1/2 tsp natural sweetener like stevia
1/2 tsp fresh, minced ginger or ground ginger
1 tsp white vinegar
Salt and pepper
Fried egg, (optional)

Instructions

Brown ground meat in 1 Tbsp of sesame oil until cooked through and no longer pink, and season with salt and pepper to taste. Remove from pan and set aside. Heat remaining sesame oil and sauté garlic, onions, and slaw in sesame oil until cabbage is cooked to desired tenderness. Stir in the soy sauce, sriracha sauce, sweetener, ginger, and vinegar. Add ground meat back in. Mix well and top with additional sliced green onion and sriracha sauce if you like it spicy. A fried egg goes great on top to complete this dish!

4 servings.

Gluten Free. Low Carb. Keto.

LOW CARB CHICKEN PAD THAI

Try this healthy hack on a Thai takeout favourite but without bringing back all the extra carb calories to your pad.

Ingredients

3 Tbsp fish sauce
1 Tbsp rice vinegar
1 Tbsp natural peanut butter
1 Tbsp soy sauce (gluten free if preferred)
2 Tbsp lime juice
3 drops liquid stevia sweetener
1 tsp sriracha sauce
1 package konjac or shirataki noodles

1 lb chicken breast, cut into bite sized pieces
2 eggs, beaten
1/2 Tbsp ginger, minced
2 cloves garlic, minced
3 large scallions, thinly sliced,
1 1/2 cups bean sprouts
2 Tbsp of sesame oil for cooking
1 lime

Toppings 1/4 cup peanuts, chopped 1/3 cup cilantro leaves, lime wedge

Instructions

Thinly slice scallions, keeping whites and greens separated. Peel and mince ginger and garlic. Roughly chop cilantro leaves. Butterfly the chicken breast then cut into small bite sized pieces. In a small bowl, whisk together all sauce ingredients until well combined and smooth. Heat sesame oil in a large pan over medium-high heat. Add ginger and garlic and stir fry until fragrant, about 30 seconds. Add scallion whites and 1 tsp sriracha sauce to pan with ginger and garlic and continue stir frying until scallions have softened, about 2-3 minutes. Once scallions have softened, add chicken to pan with the ginger, garlic, scallions, and sriracha sauce. Stir fry chicken for 5 minutes or until lightly browned and cooked through. While chicken cooks, beat 2 eggs until well combined. In a colander, drain and rinse konjac noodles thoroughly under cold water for about 2 minutes. Once chicken has finished, remove the chicken from the pan and set aside. Add noodles to the pan and stir fry noodles until warm, about 5-7 minutes.

Once noodles have warmed, add the beaten eggs to the pan with the noodles and stir fry for 2-3 minutes until the eggs have cooked. Stir frequently to break up/scramble the eggs. Once eggs have cooked, add the chicken stir fry, pad Thai sauce, and bean sprouts to the pan. Continue stir frying for about 2 minutes until all ingredients are well combined. Top with scallion greens, crushed peanuts, cilantro, and a wedge of lime to serve.

2 servings.

Gluten Free. Low Carb. Keto.

LOW CARB ITALIAN FETTUCCINE ALFREDO

It's a metabolic miracle! Enjoy a fitter Fettuccine Alfredo, still with a classic cream sauce by using low carb konjac or shirataki noodles.

Ingredients

2 Italian sausages
1/4 cup Parmesan cheese
1 package konjac or shirataki noodles
2 Tbsp butter

1/4 cup heavy cream
1 tsp dried parsley
1 tsp of garlic powder
Salt and pepper, to taste

Instructions

In a colander, drain and rinse konjac noodles thoroughly under cold water for about 2 minutes. Cook the noodles in a pan for 5-10 minutes to completely dry them. (Drying the noodles out is a key step in getting the sauce to stick to the noodles.) Cook the Italian sausages on medium heat until cooked through. Remove from heat and set aside. In the same pan the sausages were cooked in, add cream and butter. Scrape the bottom of the pan to get all the flavour from the sausages incorporated into the sauce. After cream and butter are up to temperature, add the parsley and cheese. Mix thoroughly until cheese is fully melted. Add noodles into the sauce and toss to coat. Slice cooked sausages and place atop the noodles. Top with additional Parmesan cheese and sprinkle with parsley.

2 servings.

Gluten Free. Low Carb. Keto.

BELL PEPPER NACHOS

Ring the bell as your crowd goes wild! This food fight for a more nutritious and delicious nacho night is won by these Bell Pepper Nachos.

Ingredients

4 bell peppers, cut into small wedges
1 lb ground beef or ground sausage
3 Tbsp extra-virgin olive oil
1/2 tsp ground cumin
1/2 tsp chili powder
1/4 tsp garlic powder
Salt and pepper, to taste
1 1/2 cup shredded Tex-Mex cheese
Toppings: guacamole, salsa, sour cream, hot banana peppers

Instructions

Preheat oven to 425°F and line a large baking sheet with parchment paper. Add 1 Tbsp of olive oil to frying pan. Add ground beef or sausage, breaking it up as it cooks. Cook for about 10 minutes over medium-high heat, or until cooked through. Move cooked ground beef or sausage to a plate. Spread out peppers cut side up. Toss peppers with olive oil, cumin, chili powder, garlic powder, salt and pepper. Bake peppers in oven until crisp-tender, about 10 minutes. Remove peppers from oven and top with ground beef or sausage and shredded cheese. Bake until cheese is bubbly brown, about 10 minutes.

Top with guacamole, salsa, sour cream, and hot peppers.

4 servings.

Gluten Free. Low Carb. Keto.

CREAMY CHEDDAR BEEF ENCHILADAS

The key to authentic and amazing Enchiladas is the sauce and the mix of Mexican spices. This sauce is so good and easy, you'll never reach for the store-bought stuff (with all the extra processed ingredients) again! But you will probably reach for seconds.

Enchilada Sauce

Ingredients

3 Tbsp olive oil
3 Tbsp flour (gluten-free flour if preferred)
1 Tbsp ground chili powder
1 tsp ground cumin
1/2 tsp garlic powder
1/4 tsp dried oregano

1/4 tsp salt, to taste
2 Tbsp tomato paste or tomato sauce
2 cups vegetable or beef broth
1 tsp apple cider vinegar or white vinegar
Freshly ground black pepper, to taste

Instructions

This sauce comes together quickly once you get started, so measure the dry ingredients: flour, chili powder, cumin, garlic powder, oregano and salt, into a small bowl and place it near the stove. Place the tomato paste and broth near the stove as well. In a medium-sized pot over medium heat, warm the oil until it's hot enough that a light sprinkle of the flour/spice mixture sizzles on contact. This might take a couple of minutes, so be patient and don't step away from the stove! Once it's ready, pour in the flour and spice mixture. While whisking constantly, cook until fragrant and slightly deepened in colour, about 1 minute. Whisk the tomato paste into the mixture, then slowly pour in the broth while whisking constantly to remove any lumps. Raise heat to medium-high and bring the mixture to a simmer, then reduce heat as necessary to maintain a gentle simmer.

Cook, whisking often, for about 5 to 7 minutes, until the sauce has thickened a bit and a spoon encounters some resistance as you stir. (The sauce will thicken some more as it cools.) Remove from heat, then whisk in the vinegar and season to taste with a generous amount of freshly ground black pepper. Add more salt to taste, if necessary. Now time to rock, wrap, and roll up your enchiladas!

Enchiladas

1 lb lean ground beef
1/4 onion, finely chopped
1 tsp chili powder
1 tsp ground cumin
1/2 tsp garlic powder
1/4 tsp dried oregano
1/4 tsp salt and pepper, to taste
6 soft corn (gluten-free) or low-carb tortillas
1 1/2 cups shredded cheddar cheese

Preheat the oven to 400°F. Grease a 9x13-inch baking dish with butter or oil. In 12-inch non-stick skillet, cook beef over medium-high heat 5 to 7 minutes, stirring occasionally, until thoroughly cooked; drain if needed. Add onion and cook for another 3-5 minutes until soft, and stir in 1/2 cup of the enchilada sauce. Spread 1/2 cup of the enchilada sauce evenly in bottom of baking dish. Spread 1/4 cup beef mixture down the centre of each tortilla; sprinkle with 1 Tbsp of cheese. Wrap tortillas tightly around filling, placing seam side down in baking dish. Top with remaining enchilada sauce. Sprinkle with remaining cheese. Bake for 20 to 25 minutes or until hot and bubbly. Let stand 5 minutes and then sprinkle chopped cilantro on top before serving.

6 servings.

Gluten Free. Smart Carb.

SLOWER COOKER SHORT RIBS

Beef short ribs are not always an easy find in the meat department of your local supermarket. But if you do fine them, grab them fast and go low and slow for these tasty and tender fall-off-the-bone beef short ribs.

Ingredients

4 lbs boneless or bone-in beef short ribs, about 8 short ribs
1 onion, peeled and chopped
1 tsp salt
1 tsp black pepper
1 cup beef broth

1 cup red wine
1/4 cup Worcestershire sauce
1 Tbsp tomato paste
1 tsp garlic powder
1 Sprig fresh rosemary

Instructions

Season the short ribs with salt and pepper. Heat a large skillet over high heat. Sear the short ribs on each of the 4 sides for about 60 seconds per side. Pour the beef broth, Worcestershire sauce, garlic powder, and tomato paste into a slow cooker and stir together. Place the short ribs into the liquid in the slow cooker. Place rosemary sprig on top of meat and put the lid on. Cook on low for 6-8 hours, until meat is fall-off-the-bone tender.

4 servings.

Gluten Free. Low Carb. Keto.

THE BEST BURGER

As much as I love cooking on my backyard BBQ in summer, even year-round in Atlantic Canada. Cooking burgers over a flaming hot grill, although the most popular option for most home cooks, never produces a juicy, flavourful burger like you get at a good neighbourhood diner. Because it's what you cook and how you cook it that determines a great burger.

Here's **Five Tasty Tips to make the best burger.**

1. **Fat is Flavour.** The first step to making a great burger is using flavourful meat with just enough fat-to-meat ratio. I recommend 80/20 ground beef if you are going for pure flavour, taste, and texture, as it contains 80% meat, 20% fat, and is usually labelled as lean ground beef or chuck in your supermarket. Extra lean ground beef, as it's commonly labeled, or ground sirloin or ground meat from wild or grass fed animals is usually leaner, around 90/10, 90% meat to 10% fat. It also has a more meaty, rich, beef flavour, but with less fat it can give you a drier burger, especially if cooked over open flame.

2. **Delicate not Dense.** Form loosely packed patties. Ground meat is a deceptively delicious but delicate thing. Too much woman or manhandling, and you'll ruin the amazing, tender texture that a good burger should have. So resist the urge to mix and mold the meat too much with your hands, as this isn't pottery class! And also, don't pack it with all the common fillers of onions, garlic, breadcrumbs and Worcestershire sauce, like you would with making a meatloaf. All this can make the burger patty denser and is simply more work. Instead, carefully dab each portion of meat with about a teaspoon of olive oil, then gently squeeze flat and pat the portions into a 1-inch thick patty that's approximately the diameter and thickness of your palm, or around 6 ounces. Again, don't bully the beef and push too hard or slap it around! A juicy tender burger needs some tender love and care.

3. **Simple Seasoning.** For seasoning beef and burgers, I believe the classic combo of some good coarse salt and freshly ground black pepper is all that is needed. A good layer of salt will also aid in creating a charred crust as your burger cooks. And that's what we're looking for in the best burger: a charred

crust. So here's how you correctly season a burger: Find a nice, rough-grained kosher salt or sea salt and a black pepper grinder. Now season the entire side of your patty with salt and freshly ground black pepper. Don't be shy, especially with the salt, you want good coverage. Season, flip, and repeat on the other side.

Flat not Fire. This is the absolute key to the best burger at home. Use a preheated, hot cast iron skillet. A cast iron pan is the best method for cooking a burger at home, as it's similar to the large, flat-top griddle that most diners use for great burgers and breakfasts because of the material properties of iron, plus the thickness and shape of the pan. Iron retains heat a lot better than copper or aluminum pans, and the shape of a pan itself holds all the fat and juices in as the burgers cook, opposed to an open flame BBQ where the juices and fat drip out, leaving you with flame and flare-ups. Using a cast iron pan will also help you avoid burning the burgers on the outside and drying them out on the inside. Iron takes longer to heat than other pans, but it's well worth the wait.

So, before you start preparing the patties, place a clean cast iron skillet into a 350-degree oven or on a closed-lid BBQ (if you want to still enjoy cooking outdoors on your grill). Let the pan heat thoroughly for about 15 minutes, then, when ready to cook, move it over a medium-high raised coil top burner or keep on the BBQ grill.

Warning #1: Do not use a cast iron skillet on a glass stove top, as it can permanently scratch your stove top!

Warning #2: Be extra careful when handling a hot iron skillet, as the handle will also get very hot!

Use thick oven mitts to pick up your pan, and make sure not to touch the handle without using them. I like to turn the handle away from me on the grill to resist the urge to touch it. Finally, add a tablespoon of avocado oil to the pan. Avocado oil has a higher smoke point than olive oil. If it beads slightly and shines as it hits the pan, it's ready. Don't overcrowd the pan with burgers or you will lose some heat, so for a large cast iron pan, add no more than 4 burgers; for a small pan, 2 burgers max.

5. **Patience not Pressing**. Once the burgers hit the searing hot pan, give them, and yourself, a break, and leave them alone for awhile. You want to create that charred crust that creates flavour and that requires heat and time. Resist the urge to look like you are a busy chef by constantly pressing, poking, or prodding the burgers. Once the burgers begin to show half browning on the bottom and a few red juice bubbles on top, approximately 5-7 minutes on one side, flip gently one time with a spatula. Always gently flip burgers, or any hot food cooked in a pan with grease, *away from you,* to prevent hot grease from splattering towards you and burning you. This cast iron, hot-pan sear is the ultimate key to a great burger at home—a thick charred crust that you cannot achieve the same on an open-flame grill or regular pan.

BOSTON LETTUCE–STUFFED BOCCONCINI BURGER

"Lett-uce" surprise your backyard guests with this tasty twist on a low-carb cheeseburger, and they will never miss the traditional bread bun.

Ingredients

1 lb of lean ground beef
1/2 tsp salt
1/2 tsp pepper

4 small bocconcini mozzarella balls or cubed mozzarella
1 Tbsp of avocado oil
8 Boston lettuce leaves

Instructions

Form ground beef into 4 thin, palm-size patties (to make 2 stuffed burger patties). Place a small mozzarella ball of bocconcini cheese in centre of one patty. Place other patty on top and form and press meat around cheese ball in the shape of a sealed burger patty around centre and edge, leaving no exposed cheese. Sprinkle with salt and pepper. Place patties in a preheated hot pan with avocado oil to get a good sear, and cook 5-7 minutes on each side or until juices run clear. Wash, rinse, and then pat dry lettuce leaves with paper towel and stack 2 leaves for the bottom of each burger "bun" and two leaves for the top. And extra servings of napkins!

2 servings.

Gluten Free. Low Carb. Keto.

ITALIAN MARINARA MEAT LOAF

There is no rushing a savoury meatloaf for dinner. But with this low-carb hack on a culinary classic, using almond flour and Parmesan cheese instead of the typical breadcrumbs, the smell, and then taste, will have your family "meating" you at the table for more.

Ingredients

2 lbs ground beef
1 small onion, finely chopped
1 tsp garlic powder
1 egg
1 Tbsp low-sugar ketchup
1 Tbsp mustard
1/2 cup almond flour

1/2 cup grated Parmesan cheese
1/2 cup old cheddar cheese, diced into small cubes
2 Tbsp oregano
1/2 tsp salt
1/2 tsp pepper
1 cup marinara sauce for topping

Instructions

Preheat your oven to 375ºF. In a large bowl, mix the ground beef, almond flour, Parmesan, onion, garlic powder, egg, oregano, ketchup, mustard, salt and pepper. Work the cheese cubes into the meat mixture. Line a large baking sheet with parchment paper (the baking sheet gives you more room to remove and slice than a loaf pan), then form the meatloaf with your hands into a typical rectangle meatloaf shape. Pour the marinara sauce across the top of the meatloaf. Bake until cooked through, around 60 minutes.

4 servings.

Gluten Free. Low Carb. Keto.

GO-TO GOULASH

This weeknight meal was a staple for many families growing up, including mine. Whether you had the hamburger meal in a box or your own go-to ground beef, sauce, and noodle mixture, which we called goulash. Which was a faster, Americanized version of the authentic goulash recipe of beef stew and root vegetables seasoned with paprika that originated from Hungary. This version is a cheap, classic comfort dish to feed the family fast, with so many different protein, produce, and pasta options you can play with, so the kids won't "gou-lash" out at you when they are "Hungary."

Ingredients

1 lb lean ground beef
1 small onion, chopped
1 medium bell pepper, chopped
1 cup of white button mushrooms, chopped
2 cups uncooked elbow macaroni (gluten free if preferred)
1 bottle of your favourite tomato or marinara pasta sauce
2 Tbsp of extra virgin olive oil
Salt and pepper, to taste
1 tsp of garlic powder
1 tsp of Italian seasoning
1 cup of grated cheddar cheese

Instructions

Fill a large pot 3/4 full with water. Add 1 Tbsp of salt to water. Cover and bring to a boil over high heat. Set a colander in the sink for draining the pasta. When the water reaches a boil, add the pasta. Stir with a wooden spoon for about 30 seconds, then stir occasionally while the pasta cooks. In a large non-stick frying pan, heat the oil over medium heat. Add the onion. Cook, stirring frequently with a wooden spoon until the onion is soft, about 3 minutes. Cook, stirring frequently, until soft and aromatic. Add the ground beef, salt, pepper, garlic powder, and Italian seasoning and cook, breaking up the clumps with a wooden spoon or heatproof spatula, until thoroughly cooked and browned, about 5-7 minutes. If desired, remove and discard any excess fat.

Stir the tomato sauce into the beef. Reduce heat to low. Taste. Season with salt and pepper if needed. (This is a good time to check the pasta if you haven't already.)

After about 8 minutes of boiling, check the pasta for doneness to al-dente so it doesn't overcook and get mushy. Drain the pasta in the colander and return pasta to the cooking pot. Add the meat sauce to the pasta and stir with a wooden spoon to combine. If using cheese, add it one handful at a time, stirring between each addition until the cheese is melted. Or you could choose to place the pasta and meat sauce in a casserole dish, cover the top with cheese, and broil for 5 minutes in the oven until brown and bubbly.

You can change up this easy eating meal weekly by trying ground chicken, ground turkey, or ground sausage instead of ground beef. Try other pasta options like penne, fusilli, or spaghetti. You can lower the carbs by using just 1 cup of pasta instead of 2 cups, and you will never notice the difference. Add other vegetables like spinach or broccoli. Or try different cheeses like mozzarella, goat cheese, or Parmesan works well too.

4 servings.

*Gluten Free.

SIMPLE SPAGHETTI CARBONARA

This is my favourite pasta dish when I want to enjoy some classic comfort carbs (carb is in the name after all!) but without the common combo of pasta and tomato sauce.

Ingredients

1 pound dry spaghetti (gluten free if preferred)
2 Tbsp extra-virgin olive oil
1/2 cup pancetta or bacon, cubed or chopped
4 garlic cloves, finely chopped

2 large eggs
1 cup of grated Parmesan cheese, plus more for serving
Freshly ground black pepper
1 handful fresh flat-leaf parsley, chopped

Instructions

Prepare the sauce while the pasta is cooking to ensure that the spaghetti will be hot and ready when the sauce is finished; it is very important that the pasta is hot when adding the egg mixture, so that the heat of the pasta cooks the raw eggs in the sauce.

Bring a large pot of salted water to a boil, add the regular pasta, and cook for 8 to 10 minutes or until tender yet firm (as they say in Italian "al dente"). Drain the pasta well, reserving 1/2 cup of the starchy cooking water to use in the sauce if you wish. Meanwhile, heat the olive oil in a deep skillet over medium heat. Add the pancetta or bacon and sauté for about 3 minutes, until it is crisp and the fat is rendered.

Toss the garlic into the fat and sauté for less than 1 minute to soften. Add the hot, drained spaghetti noodles to the pan and toss for 2 minutes to coat the strands in the bacon fat. Beat the eggs and Parmesan together in a mixing bowl, stirring well to prevent lumps. Remove the pan from the heat and pour the egg/cheese mixture into the pasta, whisking quickly until the eggs thicken, but do not scramble (this is done off the heat to ensure this does not happen). Thin out the sauce with a bit of the reserved pasta water until it reaches desired consistency. Season the carbonara with freshly ground black pepper and garnish with chopped parsley.

4 servings.

*Gluten Free.

DILLY OF A PICKLE CHICKEN WINGS

If you are a fan of lip-puckering pickles, the best brine for tasty tender chicken is usually waiting bottled up in your fridge.

Ingredients

3 lbs chicken wings (approximately 12-15 wings)
3 cups dill pickle brine
2 Tbsp avocado oil
2 tsp dried dill
1 tsp garlic powder
1 tsp fresh cracked black pepper
1/2 tsp salt

Instructions

Place chicken wings in a shallow baking dish or resealable plastic bag. Pour pickle juice over the top of wings and try to ensure all chicken is submerged. Cover and refrigerate for 2, or up to 24 hours. Remove from fridge, rinse, and pat dry chicken. Preheat oven to 425°F. Place a cooling rack on top of a baking sheet and set aside. In a small bowl, whisk together oil, dill, garlic powder, salt and pepper. Pour mixture over wings and toss to coat. Place wings on cooling rack placed over prepared baking sheet (helps them brown up crispier while cooking with circulating air) and bake for 25 minutes. Turn and bake an additional 10-15 minutes or until golden brown and cooked through. Serve with ranch or dill dressing if desired.

2 servings.

Gluten Free. Low Carb. Keto.

BAKED GARLIC PARMESAN CHICKEN WINGS

Get crispy coated wings baked in the oven with the secret ingredient: "baking" powder.

Ingredients

3 lbs chicken wings (approximately 12-15 wings)
2 Tbsp avocado oil
1 1/2 Tbsp baking powder
Salt and pepper
1/4 cup salted butter

4 cloves garlic, minced
2 tsp dried parsley
Pinch of red pepper flakes
1/2 cup grated Parmesan
Fresh chopped rosemary or parsley

Instructions

Preheat oven to 425°F. Pat wings dry very well with paper towel and place wings in a plastic bag. Pour in oil and move wings around to coat. Sprinkle wings with baking powder, salt, and pepper and seal the bag. Shake to coat. Place wings on cooling rack placed over prepared baking sheet (helps them brown up crispier while cooking with circulating air), and bake 25 minutes. Turn and bake an additional 10-15 minutes or until golden brown and cooked through. Transfer cooked wings to a large bowl. Melt the butter in a microwaveable safe bowl or in a saucepan. Add the garlic, parsley, and pepper flakes. Pour over the chicken wings and sprinkle with the Parmesan. Toss well to coat. Sprinkle with chopped parsley. Sprinkle with additional salt and pepper, to taste. Serve immediately with your favourite dipping sauce.

2 servings.

Gluten Free. Low Carb. Keto.

CAVEMAN CORDEN BLEU

The classic way to make Chicken Cordon Bleu involves chicken breast, pounded until thin, layered with ham and cheese, rolled into a log, chilled, dredged in wheat flour, then egg, then breadcrumbs, then deep fried in oil. That's a lot of work! And a lot of not so healthy ingredients. Go more paleo with your poultry and choose this easy eating and cooking Caveman Cordon Bleu instead.

Ingredients

6-8 boneless, skinless chicken thighs
6-8 slices of naturally smoked ham, slices cut in half
1 cup of your favourite shredded cheese
1 cup almond flour

2 cups marinara tomato sauce, divided
1 tsp dried oregano
1/2 tsp of salt
1/2 tsp of black pepper

Instructions

Preheat oven to 400°F. Pour 1 cup of marinara sauce in bottom of a casserole dish. Place half a ham slice and sprinkle of cheese inside each chicken thigh and pinch and roll in a plate full of almond flour. Place coated chicken in dish, sprinkle with seasoning, and pour remaining sauce over chicken to coat. Bake at 400°F for 30 mins.

4 servings.

Gluten Free. Low Carb. Keto.

SUPERBOWL BUFFALO CHICKEN SPAGHETTI SQUASH

Up your game in the kitchen but slice your carbs in half with spaghetti squash and these spicy, stuffed bowls will be gone by halftime.

Ingredients

1 medium spaghetti squash
1 Tbsp extra-virgin olive oil
Salt and freshly ground black pepper
2 cups shredded rotisserie chicken
1 1/2 cups shredded cheese blend, divided
1/2 cup crumbled goat cheese or blue cheese
1/2 cup plain Greek yogurt
1/2 tsp garlic powder
1/3 cup red hot sauce, plus more for serving
Ranch or blue cheese dressing, for serving
Celery and carrot sticks

Instructions

Preheat oven to 400°F. Line a baking sheet with parchment paper. Resting the squash on a secure cutting board, cut the squash in half lengthwise from stem to tail and scrape out the seeds with a large spoon. Drizzle with olive oil and season with salt and pepper, to taste. Place squash, cut side down, onto the baking sheet. Place into oven and roast until tender, about 35-45 minutes. Remove from oven and let rest until cool enough to handle. Using a fork, scrape the flesh out to create spaghetti-like strands. Mix shredded chicken, 1 cup shredded cheese, goat cheese, Greek yogurt, garlic powder, and hot sauce into bowl with the squash. Divide mixture between hollowed out squash halves and sprinkle tops with remaining 1/2 cup shredded cheese. Transfer back to baking sheet and continue to bake for 10-15 minutes until cheese is bubbling brown. Drizzle with a little more hot sauce and ranch dressing. Serve with celery and carrot sticks.

2 servings.

Gluten Free. Low Carb

CHICKEN PRIMAVERA SPAGHETTI SQUASH BOATS

Whatever floats your boat, but spaghetti squash turns a popular pasta dish into a gluten-free, low-carb treat and less dishes to clean up!

Ingredients

- 1 medium spaghetti squash, halved, seeds removed
- 2 Tbsp extra-virgin olive oil, divided
- Kosher salt
- Freshly ground black pepper
- 1/2 small onion, chopped
- 1 bell pepper, chopped
- 1 cup grape tomatoes, halved
- 1 medium zucchini, cut into halves
- 2 cloves garlic, minced
- 1 tsp lemon juice
- 1/2 tsp Italian seasoning
- 2 cups cooked, shredded chicken
- 1 cup shredded mozzarella cheese
- 1/4 cup grated Parmesan
- Freshly chopped parsley, for garnish

Instructions

Preheat oven to 400°F. Line a baking sheet with parchment paper. Resting the squash on a secure cutting board, cut the squash in half lengthwise from stem to tail and scrape out the seeds with a large spoon. Drizzle with 1 Tbsp of olive oil and season with salt and pepper, to taste. Place squash, cut side down, onto the baking sheet. Place into oven and roast until tender, about 35-45 minutes. Remove from oven and let rest until cool enough to handle. Using a fork, scrape the flesh out to create spaghetti-like strands. Meanwhile, make primavera filling.

Primavera Filling

In a large skillet over medium heat, heat remaining Tbsp of olive oil. Add onion and pepper and cook until mostly tender, 3 to 4 minutes, then add tomatoes, zucchini, garlic, and lemon juice. Season with salt, pepper, and Italian seasoning and cook 3 to 4 minutes more. Stir in chicken and remove from heat. Divide mixture between spaghetti squash halves and stir to combine.

Top each spaghetti squash with cheese and return to oven to melt, about 5 minutes. Top with Parmesan and parsley to serve.

2 servings.

Gluten Free. Low Carb.

BBQ BEER CAN CHICKEN

The ultimate summer backyard BBQ choice to feed the team, where the chef gets to drink first but the real star of the show gets the "rub" down!

Ingredients

BBQ Chicken Rub:

2 Tbsp paprika
2 Tbsp salt
2 Tbsp ground cumin

2 Tbsp dried oregano
2 Tbsp black pepper
2 Tbsp garlic powder

For the Chicken:

1 4-lb roasting chicken
1 Tbsp olive or avocado oil

1 Regular size can of beer (12-oz, 355ml)

Instructions

For the chicken rub: In a small bowl mix all the dry ingredients together and use for the BBQ chicken.

For the chicken: Preheat your BBQ grill to medium-high heat. Rub the chicken and its cavity down with the oil. Season the chicken with spice rub mixture, remembering to season the cavity. Pour out (or drink!) half of the beer and securely sit the chicken on top of the half-full beer can. Place the chicken on the grill and spread out the legs to form a secure tripod, to keep the chicken stable. Cook the chicken over medium-high, indirect heat (i.e. no coals or burners directly under the chicken). With the grill cover closed, cook the chicken for 1 to 1 1/2 hours, or until an instant-read thermometer registers 165°F. Once cooked, cover loosely with foil and let rest for 10 minutes before carving.

4 servings.

Gluten Free. Low Carb. Keto.

SUMMER SAVORY ROAST CHICKEN WITH APPLES AND ONIONS

My favourite way to use up extra apples in the fall season after apple picking with my family. The combination of the onions, summer savory, red apples and red wine melts into an aromatic, dark gravy that will make your kitchen smell as good as this roast chicken tastes, for a "savoury" Sunday dinner in any season.

Ingredients

1 4-lb roasting chicken
4 red apples, cored and quartered
2 onions, peeled and quartered
1 whole head of peeled garlic cloves
2 tsp of dried summer savory

1/2 cup of red wine
1 tsp of salt
1 tsp of pepper
2 green onions, thinly sliced

Instructions

Preheat your oven to 350°F. Toss the apples, onions, garlic, and summer savory together in a large roasting pan to hold the chicken. Season chicken with salt and pepper and rest it on top of the apple mixture. Pour in the wine. Roast chicken until a meat thermometer inserted in the thickest part of one of the thighs reads 180°F, about 20 minutes per pound, or generally 1 hour 15 minutes. As soon as the chicken is cool enough to handle, and without removing it from the pan, slice and pull the meat from the carcass and toss with the aromatic apple pan stew. Sprinkle over the sliced green onions and serve directly out of the pan to plate.

4 servings.

Gluten Free. Low Carb. Keto.

ROASTED HOLIDAY HERB TURKEY

Be the host that can "roast" before the toast to a perfect holiday turkey, and make memories around your dining room table that people will be talking about all year long.

Ingredients

1 10-15 lb fresh turkey
4 onions, peeled and halved
4 large carrots
4 stalks celery

1/2 stick butter, melted
2 tsp of salt
3 tsp of pepper

Holiday Herb Gravy

3 cups water or chicken broth
1 cup wine (any kind)
2 Tbsp cornstarch

1 Tbsp minced fresh thyme, tarragon, or rosemary
Salt and pepper

Instructions

Preheat oven to 400°F. Thoroughly pat dry the turkey with paper towels. Remove any excess moisture and dry out the skin so that it will brown well. With the onions, carrots, and celery, form a bed in the roasting pan for the turkey to rest on. Brush or rub down the turkey thoroughly with the melted butter. Season with salt and pepper. Roast turkey for 1 hour at 400°F to brown it on the outside and slowly roast on the inside to keep it moist, and then, without opening the oven, turn the heat down to 300°F and continue roasting for 2 to 3 hours longer, depending on the size of the turkey. Continue roasting until the breast and thigh meat have both reached at least 170°F. As a rough guideline, you can plan on about 12 minutes cooking time for each pound of turkey.

When done, remove from oven and cover the turkey with foil and let rest for 20 to 30 minutes before carving to give the juices inside the meat a chance to calm down and evenly redistribute themselves throughout the turkey.

Gravy

Pour off most of any accumulated fat, carefully reserving the juices. Add the liquid of your choice to the pan, along with the wine and any reserved juices, scraping the bottom of the pan to dissolve all of the browned bits. Pour all the liquid into a small saucepan, scraping every last bit of flavour out of the pan. Bring it to a simmer. Dissolve the cornstarch in a splash of water and add to the pan, whisking until the gravy thickens. Whisk in some fresh herbs, then taste, season, and enjoy!

8 servings.

Gluten Free. Low Carb. Keto.

CHICKEN MARINARA MEATBALLS

Ingredients

Roll on over beef, these chicken marinara meat balls are so "clucking" good, you'll never call them meatballs again, I "swear!"

2 lbs ground chicken
1 egg
1/2 cup almond flour
1/2 cup grated Parmesan
2 Tbsp olive oil

1/2 teaspoon garlic powder
1/2 teaspoon dried oregano
Salt and black pepper, to taste
1 cup marinara sauce

Instructions

Preheat the oven to 400°F. Line a baking sheet with parchment paper. Mix all the ingredients, except marinara sauce, together in a mixing bowl. With wet hands, roll the mixture into golf ball-size chicken balls. Place on baking sheet, leaving a little space between them. Bake for 25-30 minutes. Pour marinara sauce over chicken balls during the last 10 minutes of cooking.

Yields 12-15 meatballs.

4-6 servings.

Gluten Free. Low Carb. Keto.

CAMPFIRE MEATBALL ONION BOMBS

These fun and flavourful foil-wrapped meatballs are always a hit around the campfire or backyard fire pit on a warm summer's night. These meatballs are, as the kids say, "da-bomb!"

Ingredients

3 large onions
2 lbs lean ground beef
1 egg
1/2 cup almond flour
1/2 cup grated Parmesan

2 Tbsp olive oil
1/2 teaspoon garlic powder
1/2 teaspoon dried oregano
Salt and black pepper, to taste
1 cup marinara sauce or ketchup

Instructions

Peel large onions and cut in half. Separate the onions into matching pieces to make thin C-shaped casings to wrap around each side of each meatball. In a bowl, using wet hands, mix together all the remaining meatball ingredients except for the marinara sauce. Do not over mix the meat, or the meatballs will become too dense. Press each onion slice around each side of a meatball and press it together. Repeat. Wrap 5 or 6 meatball onion bombs per foil packet. (I recommend heavy duty aluminum foil and wrap at least 2 times.) To cook, place foil-wrapped packets around the edges of a campfire with very hot coals for 15-20 minutes. Flip over with long BBQ tongs and cook for another 15-20 minutes. Total cooking time will depend on the size of your meatballs and the heat of your coals. Check on them to be sure they are cooked all the way through. You can also roast these in a 350ºF oven or atop a closed BBQ grill. To serve, using tongs, oven mitts, or gloves, remove the foil packets from the fire, open to allow steam to escape, and top with warmed marinara sauce or ketchup if desired.

Yields 12-15 meatballs.

4-6 servings.

Gluten Free. Low Carb.

STEAKHOUSE SKILLET CHEESEBURGER MEATBALLS

Ingredients

2 lbs lean ground beef
1 egg
1/2 cup almond flour
1/2 cup grated Parmesan
2 Tbsp olive oil
1/2 teaspoon garlic powder

1/2 teaspoon dried oregano
Salt and black pepper, to taste
1 Tbsp water
3 Tbsp steak sauce
5 slices thin pre-sliced old cheddar cheese, each cut in 4 small squares

Instructions

Mix all the ingredients, except the cheese, together in a mixing bowl. With wet hands, roll the mixture into 12-15 golf ball-size meatballs. Heat a 12-inch non-stick skillet over medium heat. Add meatballs and cook 12 to 14 minutes, turning frequently to brown on all sides, to internal temperature of 160°F. Remove from heat. Add 3 tablespoons steak sauce and the water, and gently stir to coat. Top each meatball with a small cheese square and cover pan for 1 to 2 minutes or until cheese melts. Insert toothpick in each meatball and serve. Yields 12-15 meatballs.

4-6 servings.

Gluten Free. Low Carb.

CILANTRO LIME CHARRED CHICKEN THIGHS

Juicy, tender grilled chicken bursting with citrusy, fiery flavours that can be topped or chopped over rice, tacos, or salads, for a winner winner chicken dinner.

Ingredients

6-8 boneless, skinless chicken thighs
1/4 cup chopped, fresh cilantro leaves
3 Tbsp extra-virgin olive oil, divided
2 Tbsp freshly squeezed lime juice

2 tsp chili powder
1 tsp ground cumin
1 tsp kosher salt
1 tsp freshly ground black pepper

Instructions

In a medium bowl, combine cilantro, 2 tablespoons olive oil, lime juice, chili powder, cumin, salt and pepper. In a large size resealable bag or large bowl, combine chicken and cilantro marinade mixture and place bag on a plate in the fridge. Marinate for at least 1 hour to overnight, turning the bag occasionally. When ready to cook, remove the chicken from the marinade. Grease BBQ grill with avocado oil and preheat to 400°F for 5-10 minutes. Add chicken thighs to hot grill and don't try to turn them over until they release easily from the grill in order to get golden grill marks and develop a nice char on the outside. (If it sticks it's not ready to flip!) You can also cook the chicken in a hot, oiled pan if needed. Cook until golden brown on both sides and cooked through, reaching an internal temperature of 165°F, about 10 minutes per side. Once done, let the cooked chicken rest for 5-10 minutes allowing juices to redistribute.

4 servings.

Gluten Free. Low Carb. Keto.

GARLIC BUTTER BAKED CHICKEN THIGHS & BABY POTATOES

This tasty twist on chicken and potatoes is a one and done dinner in 30 minutes and will impress everyone from "babies" to adults.

Ingredients

6-8 boneless, skinless chicken thighs
Salt and pepper
1/2 cup or (1 stick) garlic butter, softened to room temperature
1 Tbsp lemon juice
1 Tbsp dried thyme
1 lemon, cut into rounds
1 lb baby potatoes, quartered
1 Tbsp freshly chopped parsley, for garnish

Instructions

Preheat oven to 425°F. Season chicken all over with salt and pepper. In a medium bowl, stir together garlic butter, lemon juice, and thyme. Mix garlic butter all over chicken thighs and potatoes. Place lemon rounds on bottom of baking dish, then layer potatoes and chicken thighs, and bake until thighs register 160°F on an instant-read thermometer, about 30 minutes. Top with chopped parsley.

4 servings.

Gluten Free. Smart Carb.

TASTY TURKEY CHILI

You won't be asking yourself, "Where's the beef?" once you try this leaner and lighter chili that always warms up a crowd on game day.

Ingredients

2 tsp olive oil
1 yellow onion, chopped
1 medium red bell pepper, chopped
1 lb extra lean ground turkey
2 Tbsp chili powder
2 tsp garlic powder
2 tsp ground cumin
1 tsp dried oregano
1/4 tsp cayenne pepper

1/2 tsp salt and pepper, plus more, to taste
2 (28-oz) cans diced tomatoes
1 (15 oz) can dark red kidney beans, rinsed and drained OR
(*low carb and low FODMAP option) replace beans with 1 cup finely diced carrots

For toppings: cheese, avocado, corn tortilla chips, cilantro, sour cream

Instructions

Place oil in a large pan and place over medium-high heat. Add in onion and red pepper and sauté for 5-7 minutes, stirring frequently. Add in ground turkey and break up the meat, cooking until no longer pink. Next, add in chili powder, cumin, oregano, cayenne pepper, and salt. Stir for about 30 seconds. Next, in a separate, large pot, add in canned tomatoes and kidney beans (or chopped carrots.) Add cooked turkey to pot of tomatoes and bring to a boil. Reduce heat and simmer for 30-45 minutes or until chili thickens and flavours come together. Taste and adjust seasonings and salt as necessary. Garnish with listed toppings if you desire.

6-8 servings.

Gluten Free. Smart Carb.

SAUCY STUFFED CABBAGE ROLLS

It seems we all have one family or friend who makes great cabbage rolls. Now you can be one of them with some easy eating tips and tricks. Even better, they freeze well and taste better the next day, should you be lucky enough to have any leftovers!

Ingredients

2 lbs of lean ground beef
1 head green savoy cabbage
1 pkg of microwave instant white rice
3 garlic cloves, minced
1/2 medium onion, chopped
1 tsp dry basil
1 tsp dry oregano
1/2 tsp garlic powder

Sauce

2 (28-oz) cans crushed or diced tomatoes
1 garlic clove, crushed

Mix sauce ingredients

Ingredients

Preheat oven to 350°F. Wash and cut bottom stem out of cabbage. Boil head of cabbage and gradually remove leaves with tongs while boiling (they should fall off easily). In a frying pan, add garlic, onions, and herbs, and sauté on medium for 2-3 minutes. Add ground beef and pre-cooked microwaved rice. Cut bottom stem out of each cabbage leaf in a V pattern. Add half of the tomato sauce into the meat and rice mixture and stir. Add a spoonful of the meat filling to the centre of the cabbage leaf. Starting at the stem end, begin to roll while tucking in both sides. Place roll in the casserole dish seam side down. Repeat with the other cabbage leaves—you should end up with about 10-12 rolls. Pour the remaining tomato sauce over top of your cabbage rolls and bake in the oven for 1 hour. For a lower carb option, substitute riced cauliflower for white rice.

6 servings.

Gluten Free.

HEALTHY HOT DOG

"Frankly" it's best you ditch the mystery meat and soggy-bun hot dog at the ball park or street corner and try this healthy hack on a hot dog that is sure to be a hit at your "home plate."

Ingredients

1 Fit and Fast Flaxseed Wrap
1 bratwurst or favourite gluten-free sausage

Toppings:

1 Tbsp chopped onion
1 Tbsp hot banana peppers
1 Tbsp sauerkraut

1 Tbsp ketchup
1 Tbsp yellow mustard

Instructions

Prepare Fit and Fast Flaxseed Wrap located in this book and let it cool. Heat lightly greased BBQ grill or skillet to medium heat and cook sausage 5-7 minutes on both sides until golden brown or until juices run clear. (Use tongs to turn, not a fork.) Place 1 sausage on flax wrap and cover with classic suggested hot dog toppings.

1 serving.

Gluten Free. Low Carb. Keto.

HONEY GARLIC CHICKEN

A tasty Thai twist chicken dinner for when you're asked, "honey what's for dinner?"

Ingredients

1/4 cup soy sauce (gluten free if preferred)
3 Tbsp honey
2 cloves garlic, minced
Juice of 1 lime
2 Tbsp sesame oil, divided
1 tsp sriracha
1 Tbsp cornstarch
1 lb boneless, skinless chicken breasts
Kosher salt, to taste
Freshly ground black pepper
Sesame seeds, for garnish
Sliced green onions, for garnish

Instructions

Preheat oven to 350°F. In a medium bowl, whisk together soy sauce, honey, garlic, lime juice, 1 tablespoon sesame oil, sriracha, and cornstarch. Season chicken with salt and pepper. In a large oven-safe skillet over medium-high heat, heat remaining tablespoon sesame oil. Add chicken and sear until golden, about 4-5 minutes per side. Pour over glaze and transfer to oven. Bake until chicken is no longer pink, around 25 minutes. Heat broiler. Spoon glaze over chicken and broil until caramelized, for 2 minutes. Garnish with green onions and sesame seeds.

4 servings.

Gluten Free. Low Carb.

CHEESESTEAK PORTOBELLO MUSHROOMS

Up the meaty mushroom taste and texture of a Philly cheesesteak while you lower the carbs, by knocking out the bun like Rocky would.

Ingredients

1 lb sirloin steak, sliced
3 Tbsp extra-virgin olive oil, divided
4 portobello mushrooms, stems and gills removed
1 onion, sliced
2 bell peppers, sliced
Salt and freshly ground black pepper, to taste
4 slices provolone or mozzarella cheese
Chopped parsley

Instructions

Preheat oven to 350°F. Brush clean mushroom caps with 1 tablespoon olive oil, season with salt and pepper, and place them stem side up on a large baking sheet lined with parchment paper. In a large skillet over medium heat, heat 1 tablespoon olive oil. Add onion and peppers and season with salt and pepper. Cook, stirring often until the vegetables are tender, about 5 minutes. Remove from heat. Add remaining olive oil to skillet and increase heat to medium-high. Season sliced steak all over with salt and pepper and cook until the steak is browned on both sides, about 3-5 minutes. Turn off heat and return vegetable mixture to the pan. Spoon the steak mixture into mushroom caps then top with cheese. Bake until the peppers are tender, and the cheese is melted, about 20 minutes. Garnish with parsley.

4 servings.

Gluten Free. Low Carb. Keto.

THE PERFECT BBQ STEAK

Be the king or queen of your grill when guests are over and the "steaks" are high, and sear and slice the perfect steak!

Ingredients

2 steaks of choice like striploin, T-bone, filet, or rib-eye
Coarse sea salt

Coarse freshly ground black pepper
Avocado oil

Instructions

Remove your steaks from the fridge for 20-30 minutes to bring them to room temperature and use a paper towel to pat dry and remove excess moisture.

Make sure to clean and coat your BBQ grill grates with a high-temperature cooking oil like avocado oil. Get your grill smoking hot. Preheat your grill for at least 10-15 minutes on high with the lid closed.

Place your prepared steaks on the BBQ grill grates. Let the first side sear. Only if the steaks release from the grill naturally, are you ready to flip them. If the sides stick, they aren't ready to turn or flip. After the first 2-3 minutes, using tongs, turn your steaks one quarter turn. This will help give them good crosshatch grill marks. Finish the crosshatch sears on those first sides for an additional 2-3 minutes. Now flip the steaks to grill the other side. Repeat the process to create crosshatch grill marks on the other side. But be careful not to overcook. Cook using an instant-read thermometer to desired doneness, or use this general guide time chart. Grill 2 to 3 minutes per side for medium-rare (an internal temperature of 135°F), 3 to 4 minutes per side for medium (140° F) or 5 to 7 minutes per side for medium-well (150°F). Don't cut the meat right after cooking it! Let it rest for 10 minutes, covered loosely with foil. Cut the meat across the grain to get the most tender slices. Do this by cutting perpendicular to the long parallel muscle fibres in the meat. Sprinkle slices with course salt to taste.

2 servings.

Gluten Free. Low Carb. Keto.

BACKUP BROIL STEAK

For the times when you go to fire up the backyard BBQ but it's out of gas, or the winter weather is just too cold to get grilling. Don't let that foil your plans, when you can broil your plans!

Ingredients

2 steaks of choice like striploin, T-bone, filet, or ribeye
Coarse sea salt

Coarse freshly ground black pepper
Avocado oil
Cast iron skillet pan

Instructions

Remove your steaks from the fridge for 20-30 minutes to bring them to room temperature and use a paper towel to pat dry and remove excess moisture. Move oven rack 6 inches from top heating element. Preheat oven and cast iron skillet by setting the oven to broiler for 15 minutes. Rub steaks with avocado oil, course salt and freshly ground pepper. Once the skillet is preheated, pull out the oven rack and carefully lay steaks on the skillet. NOTE: Pan is extremely hot and will spit and splatter! It might get a little smoky in your kitchen so turn on stove hood fan or open a window. Sear the steaks for 3 minutes on one side, then turn steaks over using tongs and sear the opposite side for 3 minutes. Once seared, set the oven to 500°F and cook using an instant-read thermometer to desired doneness. Broil 2 to 3 minutes per side for medium-rare (an internal temperature of 135°F), 3 to 4 minutes per side for medium (140° F) or 5 to 7 minutes per side for medium-well (150°F).

Using a thick oven mitt, remove hot pan and steaks from the oven. Don't cut the meat right after cooking it! Let it rest for 10 minutes, covered loosely with foil. Cut the meat across the grain to get the most tender slices. Do this by cutting perpendicular to the long parallel muscle fibres in the meat. Sprinkle slices with course salt to taste.

2 servings.

Gluten Free. Low Carb. Keto.

EASY BREEZY BEEF STEW

Have a savoury meat and vegetables dinner on the table fast with this slow cooker, easy breezy beef stew.

Ingredients

2 lbs lean stewing beef, cut into 1-inch cubes
1/4 cup almond flour
1/2 tsp sea salt
1/2 tsp freshly ground black pepper
1 clove garlic, minced
1 bay leaf
1 tsp paprika

1 Tbsp of Worcestershire sauce or red wine
1 onion, chopped
1 1/2 cups beef broth
3 red skin potatoes, diced
4 carrots, sliced
1 stalk celery, chopped

Instructions

Place meat in slow cooker. In a small bowl, mix together the flour, salt, and pepper. Pour over meat, and stir to coat meat with flour mixture. Stir in the garlic, bay leaf, paprika, Worcestershire sauce, onion, beef broth, potatoes, carrots, and celery. Cover, and cook on low setting for 8 hours or on high for 4 hours. Remove bay leaf before serving.

4 servings.

Gluten Free. Smart Carb.

LEANER LASAGNA

Go no-noodle by choosing skinny zucchini for a leaner lasagna that packs lots of fresh flavour in this classic comfort dish.

Ingredients

1 large zucchini
1 1/2 tsp salt
1 lb pound lean ground beef
3/4 tsp ground black pepper
1 tsp of garlic powder or fresh garlic
1/2 small green bell pepper, diced
1/2 onion, diced
1 bottle (907g) marinara or tomato sauce
2 Tbsp red wine

1 Tbsp chopped fresh basil
1 Tbsp chopped fresh parsley
1 tsp dried oregano
1 (500g) container ricotta or cottage cheese
1/2 cup chopped baby spinach
1/2 cup fresh mushrooms, sliced
2 cups shredded mozzarella cheese
1/4 cup grated Parmesan cheese

Instructions

Preheat oven to 325°F. Grease a deep 9x13 inch baking dish. Slice zucchini lengthwise into very thin slices using a mandolin slicer. Sprinkle slices lightly with salt and set aside to drain on a paper towel. To prepare the meat sauce, cook and stir ground beef, garlic, and black pepper in a large skillet over medium-high heat for 5-10 minutes. Add in green pepper, mushrooms, and onion. Cook and stir until meat is no longer pink. Stir in tomato sauce, wine, basil, and oregano, adding a small amount of hot water if sauce is too thick. Bring to a boil. Reduce heat and simmer sauce for about 20 minutes, stirring frequently. Meanwhile, stir ricotta, spinach, and parsley together in a bowl until well combined.

To assemble lasagna, spread 1/2 of the meat sauce into the bottom of prepared pan. Then layer 1/2 the zucchini slices, 1/2 the ricotta mixture, all of the spinach, then 1/2 the mozzarella cheese. Repeat by layering the remaining meat sauce, zucchini slices, ricotta mixture, and mozzarella. Spread Parmesan cheese evenly over the top. Cover with foil. Bake for 45 minutes. Remove foil and raise oven temperature to 350°F (175°C) and bake an additional 15 minutes. Let stand for 5 minutes before serving.

6 servings.

Gluten Free. Low Carb.

SEAFOOD

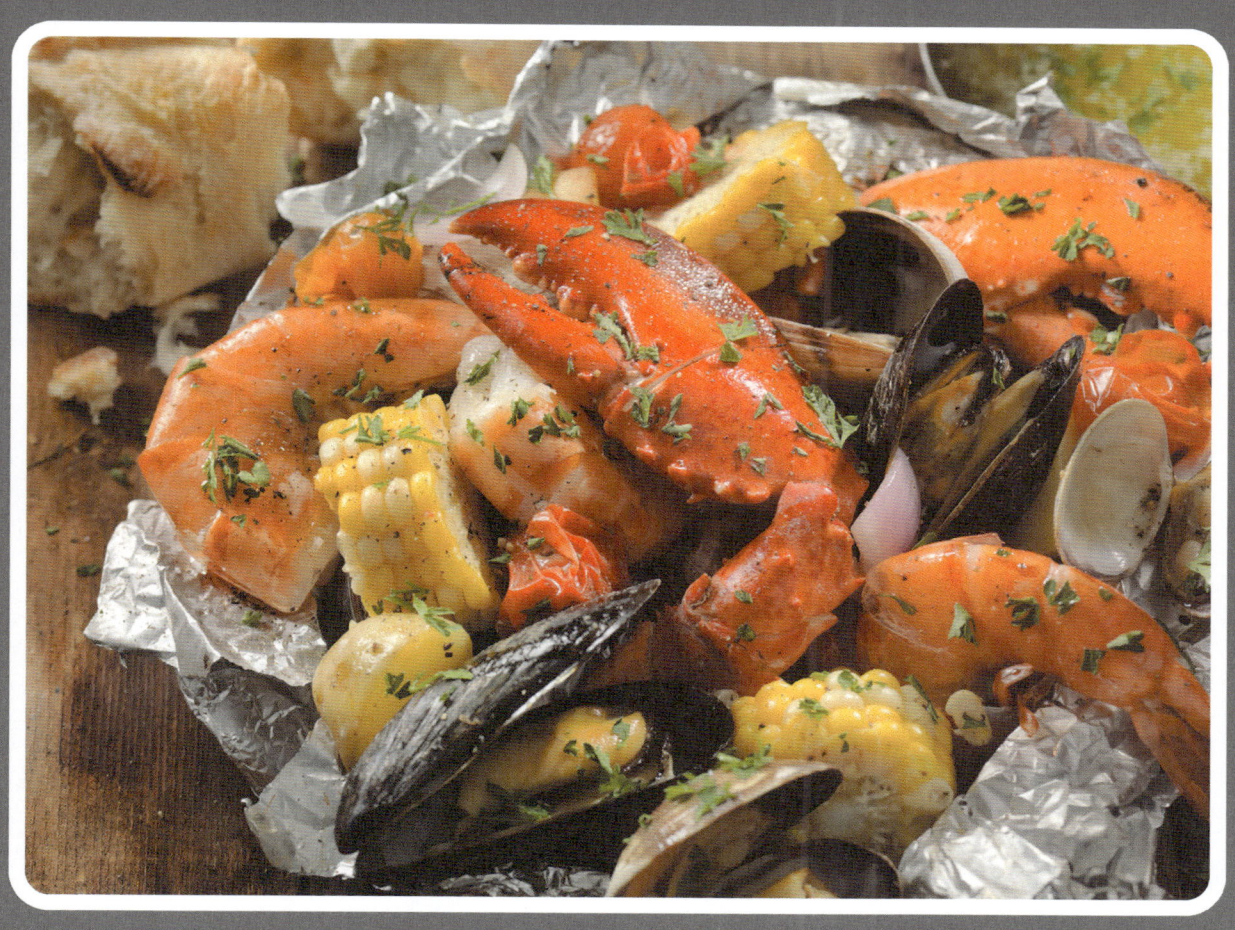

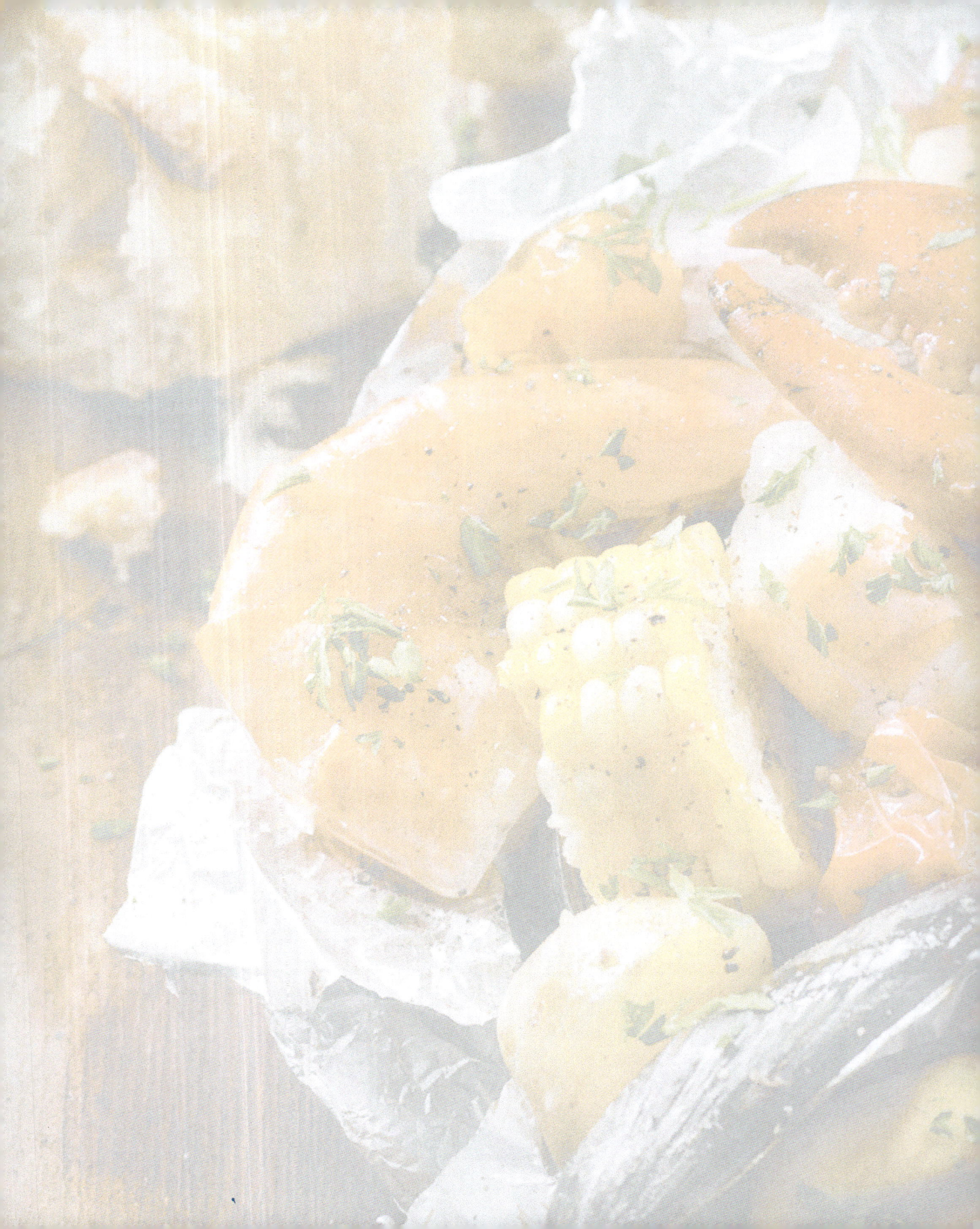

LEMON GARLIC SHRIMP

When you "see-food" with these 3 main ingredients of lemon, garlic, and shrimp, you know you have a fast and flavourful meal in minutes.

Ingredients

2 Tbsp butter, divided
1 Tbsp extra-virgin olive oil
1 lb medium shrimp, peeled and deveined
1 lemon, thinly sliced, plus juice of 1 lemon

3 cloves garlic, minced
1 tsp crushed red pepper flakes
Salt, to taste
2 Tbsp dry white wine (or water)
Freshly chopped parsley, for garnish

Instructions

In a large skillet over medium heat, melt 1 tablespoon butter and olive oil. Add shrimp, lemon slices, garlic, and crushed red pepper flakes, and season with salt. Cook, stirring occasionally, until shrimp is pink and opaque, about 3 minutes per side. Remove from heat and stir in remaining butter, lemon juice, and white wine. Season with salt and garnish with parsley before serving.

4 servings.

Gluten Free. Low Carb. Keto.

CUMIN–CRUSTED FISH

Whether you say "Q-men" or "Coo-men" for Cumin, this smoky spice adds a Cuban flavour and a crust to flaky fish that jumps to your plate in minutes.

Ingredients

1 lb white fish fillets (cod, haddock, walleye, halibut)
1 Tbsp ground cumin
1/4 tsp thyme
1 tsp paprika

1/2 tsp lemon pepper
1 Tbsp avocado oil
2 Tbsp chopped parsley
lemon or lime wedges

Instructions

In a small bowl, mix together cumin, thyme, paprika, and lemon pepper. Rub spice mixture on both sides of fillets. In a large skillet over medium heat, heat avocado oil. Add fish fillets and cook until browned on both sides and fish is opaque in the centre, about 4 minutes per side. Sprinkle with parsley and serve immediately with lemon or lime wedges.

4 servings.

Gluten Free. Low Carb. Keto.

NO-FUSS FOIL-WRAPPED BBQ SALMON

No fishy smell in your house and no messy pans or cleanup with this no-fuss foil-wrapped BBQ salmon.

Ingredients

4 boneless salmon fillets with skin on
1 small bunch of fresh dill, divided
1 medium lemon, plus additional for serving

2 Tbsp melted unsalted butter
3 cloves minced garlic
3/4 tsp kosher salt
1/4 tsp freshly ground black pepper

Instructions

Preheat an outdoor grill to medium (about 375°F). Set out a piece of aluminum foil about twice the size of each piece of salmon. Arrange a few sprigs of fresh dill down the middle of the foil. Cut the lemons into thin slices and arrange half of the slices down the middle with the dill. Place a salmon filet on top, skin side down. Drizzle the salmon with the melted butter. Sprinkle with the salt and pepper. Scatter the garlic over the top, then lay a few more springs of dill and the remaining lemon slices on top of the salmon. Fold the sides of each piece of aluminum foil up and over the top of the salmon until it is completely enclosed and forms a sealed packet. Leave a little room inside the foil for air to circulate. Carefully slide the wrapped salmon packets onto the grill. Close the grill and grill the salmon for 12-14 minutes, until the salmon is almost completely cooked through at the thickest part. When you can insert a fork into the fillet and it's warm and flaky, it should be done. Remove from grill, open the packets and let steam out as not to overcook. Slide a spatula underneath the fillet between the skin and the flesh. It should slide right off the skin.

4 servings.

Gluten Free. Low Carb. Keto.

SIMPLY STEAMED MUSSELS

High in protein, omega-3 healthy fats, and zinc, mussels are good for your muscles and pop open in the pot in just minutes! A crowd pleaser after a day at the beach, or even better, eaten at the beach.

Ingredients

2 lbs mussels, cleaned
1 Tbsp butter
2 small shallots, thinly sliced
2 garlic cloves, finely chopped
1 cup low-sodium chicken stock

1/2 cup dry white wine
1/3 cup heavy cream
1/4 cup roughly chopped fresh parsley
Salt and freshly ground black pepper
Lemon wedges, for serving

Instructions

Before you start cooking, you should always give your mussels a good rinse. Mussels should still be alive, so the fresh water rinse will cause the mussels to close. If there are any that don't close, give them a quick tap and pinch, if they still don't close, at least partially, or are broken open, simply discard them.

Melt butter over medium heat in a large pot with lid. When the butter begins to bubble, stir in the shallot and garlic. Cook until softened, about 5 minutes. Add the chicken stock, white wine, and mussels, then give them a good stir. Cover the pot with its lid and cook until all mussels have opened, 6 to 10 minutes. If any mussels still do not open, discard them. Remove the pot from the heat, then stir in the cream and parsley. Taste the broth then adjust to taste with salt, pepper, or more cream. Serve in big bowls with lemon wedges.

2 servings.

Gluten Free. Low Carb. Keto.

FINGER DIPPIN' AND LICKIN' LOBSTER

Here in New Brunswick, Canada, known as the lobster capital of the world, we take our seafood seriously. So get your "jaws" and "claws" ready for Lobster 101, because nothing tastes more like summer by the sea than freshly cooked lobster, boiled in salt water, and dipped in warm garlic butter. Mmmm lobster!

Ingredients

Lobsters
A pot large enough to hold 4 large lobsters (4-5 gallon pot)
3 gallons of water, or enough to cover lobsters

1 cup sea salt
4 large, live lobsters, roughly 1 1/2 pounds each.

Garlic Butter

1 cup butter
1 Tbsp minced garlic

2 Tbsp fresh lemon juice
1 tsp ground black pepper

Instructions

Bring a large pot of heavily salted water to a boil. The water should be salty like sea water (in fact you can use clean sea water if you have it nearby). Remove the rubber bands from the live lobster's claws by crossing over and firmly grasping their claws so they can't pinch you, then take them off. If you leave the rubber bands on while cooking, you risk getting a rubbery taste on your lobsters and I simply do not like the idea of boiling rubber with my food. Hold the lobster by the body and gently lower it headfirst into the boiling water. Bring the water back to a full boil, then lower to a simmer and set your timer for 15 minutes for four 1 1/2-pound lobsters. The lobsters should be a bright red colour when done. Note that larger lobsters will turn bright red before they are completely finished cooking, so you do want to time your cooking and not just go on colour alone. When done, remove the lobsters with tongs and place them in a colander to drain and cool.

For the Garlic Butter

Melt 1 tablespoon of butter in a saucepan over medium heat. Add the garlic; cook and stir until starting to brown, about 3 minutes. Add the remaining butter and reduce heat to low. Stir to melt the butter, then mix in the lemon juice and pepper. Let it steep over low heat for about 10 minutes. Or for easier eating and dipping if you are feeding a crowd, it's OK to buy the pre-made garlic butter at your supermarket. I won't judge.

4 servings.

Gluten Free. Low Carb. Keto.

HOW TO EAT LOBSTER

Before you get started, you'll want to assemble some easy eating essentials. You'll need a nutcracker or similar lobster claw crackers and thin lobster forks specifically designed for eating lobster. If you are stuck without those, you can get by with a large kitchen knife or cleaver, a rolling pin or hammer, or some kitchen shears and using the handle ends of some forks or spoons. A pair of rubber garden gloves helps too for grip on the wet, sharp shells to prevent cutting your hands. Best to also have a large bowl to discard the shells, a small dipping bowl for melted garlic butter, and a lot of napkins! That's why seafood restaurants give you the famous and funny plastic bibs when they serve you lobster. Eating lobster is messy but fun and one of the few foods where you can feel like a sophisticated adult and a little kid, all at the same time.

Because it can get messy, I prefer to eat fresh lobster in the summer, outdoors on a warm sunny day if possible, on a patio or picnic table if I can, and extra experience points if I am seaside and have a view of the ocean! It always brings back memories of summer vacation on the East Coast of Canada for me. Eating lobsters should be a treat that is meant to be relaxing and fun and shared with friends and families.

After the lobster cools for a few minutes, so it's not too hot to handle, start with the claws: Twist the claws away from the body at the joints that connect them to the body. Separate the knuckle from the claw. Pull back the "jaw" of the claw until it breaks, but do it gently, so that the little bit of meat that is in the small part of the claw jaw stays attached to the rest of the meat (it's easier than trying to fish it out of the small shell).

Use a nut or lobster claw cracker to crack the main claw shell. Depending on the season and the size of your lobster, the shell may be easy or hard to crack with a nutcracker. If necessary, you can take a hammer or large knife to it, but do it gently, just enough to break the shell without crushing the meat inside. Pull away the broken shell pieces and pull out the meat inside. Any white stuff attached to the meat is fat, which you can choose to eat or not, or dip into melted butter or not. Extract meat from the knuckles: Use kitchen shears (if you have them) to cut the knuckle shell along its length. Pry open the shell where you made the cut and you can pull out all the knuckle meat in one piece. Alternately, you can crack each section of knuckle with a nutcracker and pull the meat out in chunks.

If you have a very large lobster, you can eat the legs. The legs contain some sweet pieces of meat, but they pose the biggest problem in terms of removal.

An easy solution is to cut the knuckle from the top of each leg. Then, using a rolling pin, roll over each leg from the pointed tip to the open end. The meat will pop right out.

Now on to the lobster tail, where the biggest piece of meat lies. You'll need both hands to get the meat from the tail. Grip the lobster's body with one hand and the tail with the other. Bend the tail back away from the body to separate it from the body. You will see one, and maybe two, odd things inside if you are unfamiliar with lobster. You'll see the greenish tomalley, which is the lobster's liver. You can choose to eat it or not. If the lobster is a female, you may also see the bright red coral, which is the roe or tiny eggs of the lobster. You may also choose to eat this or not.

The tail will now look like a really big shrimp. Grab the flippers at the end of the tail and bend them backwards gently. If you do it right, you'll get the meat from the inside of one or more flippers. This is uncommonly sweet meat, so don't forget the morsels in the flippers. You can pry them out by working the little joints back and forth, or use shears to cut their thin shells.

With the flippers off the tail, you can now just put your finger through the small opening where the flippers were and push the big piece of tail meat out in one long piece. If you have an exceptionally large lobster, use kitchen shears to cut a line down the underside of the tail to help remove the meat. Remove the digestive tract: Before you eat the tail, pull off the top of it. This will reveal a digestive vein which you will likely want to remove, much like deveining a shrimp. It won't hurt you if you eat it, but it is the digestive tract of the lobster. There is meat inside the body of the lobster, mostly right around where you pulled off the tail. For lobsters bigger than 2 pounds, it is worth it to fish around for these extra morsels. Now just dip the meat in melted garlic butter and enjoy your feed of finger dippin' and lickin' lobster!

PIZZA

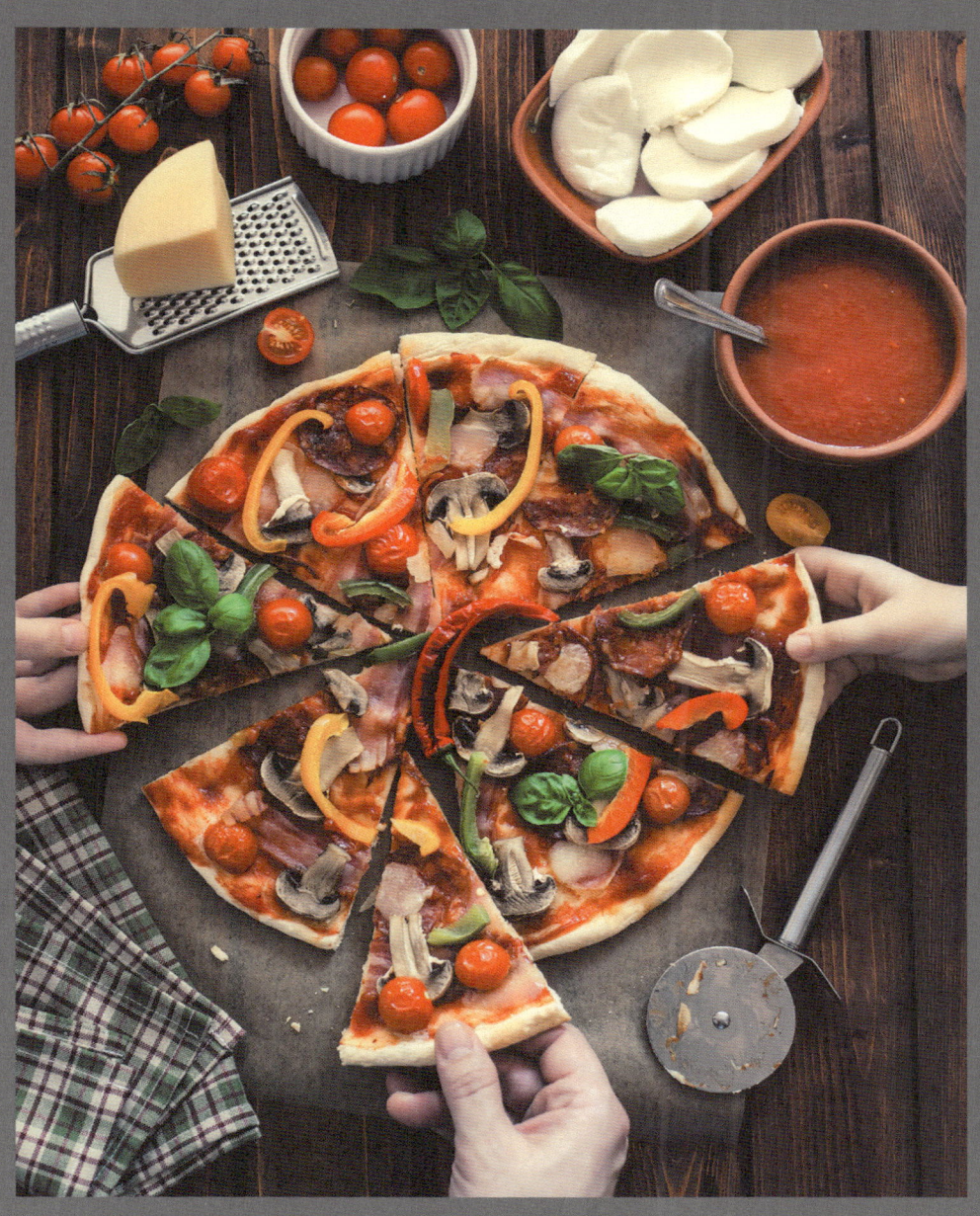

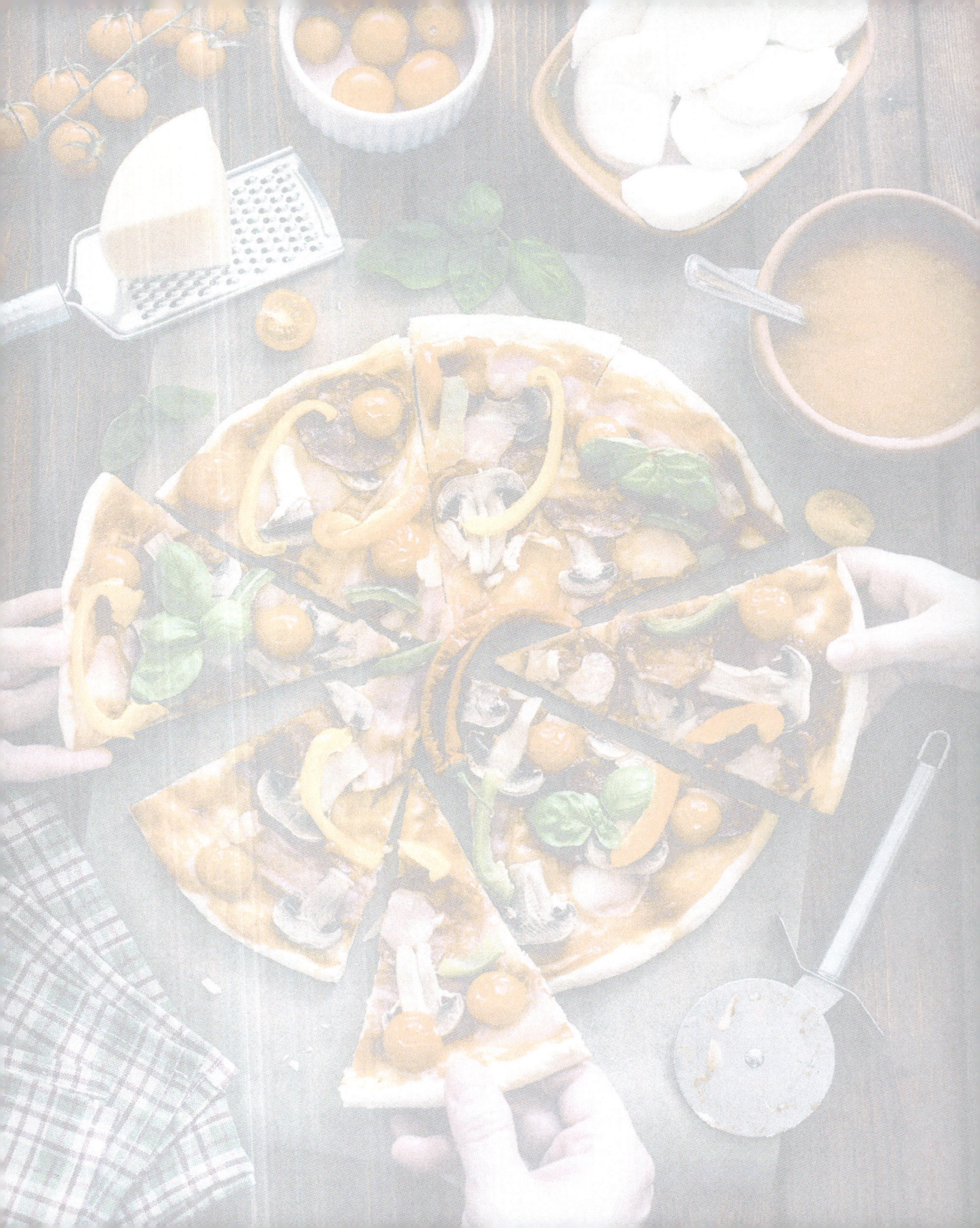

OAT FLOUR PIZZA

Pizza will always be my favourite food (it did make the cover of this book!) and this is my tried and true gluten-free homemade pizza recipe when I want to enjoy the classic pizza-making process as much as the taste and texture, using the natural flour power of oatmeal.

Ingredients

- 3 cups old fashion oats (gluten free if preferred)
- 2 1/4 tsp active dry yeast
- 2 Tbsp extra-virgin olive oil
- 1 tsp salt
- 1 1/2 Tbsp honey
- 1 cup warm water
- 2 cups marinara sauce
- 2 cups of shredded mozzarella cheese
- 2 Tbsp grated Parmesan cheese
- 1/3 cup sliced pepperoni
- 1/3 cup chopped green pepper
- 1/3 cup sliced mushrooms
- 1 Tbsp dried oregano

Instructions

Preheat oven to 375°F. To make the oat flour, place the oats in a food processor or high-powered blender and blend 1-2 minutes until a fine powder. Combine and mix the oat flour, salt, yeast, and honey in a medium sized bowl. Next, add the olive oil and water. (NOTE: The dough will be very wet and sticky at first, compared to wheat flour dough after all ingredients are mixed. Don't panic!) Add a little more olive oil or oat flour over dough and on your hands and around inside of bowl to prevent dough from sticking to your fingers and bowl, and knead the dough for 3-4 minutes, folding it over with your fingers and pressing it down with your knuckles and it will come together smoothly. It should begin to pick up all the excess dough around the bottom and sides of the bowl and resemble the texture of a big ball of smooth silly putty.

After kneading the dough until smooth and elastic, use your hands to spread the dough evenly on a pizza pan or baking sheet lined with parchment paper. Try to get the dough as spread out as possible using the tips of your fingers, without ripping the dough (I use a large pizza pan and spread the dough to cover about 90% of the pan).

Bake the crust for 10 minutes at 375°F, then remove from oven and add toppings (marinara sauce, cheese, meats, veggies, and spices). Finish baking for about 20 minutes (or until crust and cheese are golden brown). Remove pizza from oven and allow it to sit or the hot pizza pan for about 10 minutes before slicing. (Waiting for pizza to cool is always the hardest part!)

4 servings.

Gluten Free. Smart Carb.

PORTOBELLO PEPPERONI PIZZAS

You "mush make room" for this perfect pizza portion on your menu that keeps the carbs and food fuss low but the flavour and nutrients high.

Ingredients

6 large portobello mushrooms
1 Tbsp olive oil
6 Tbsp marinara tomato sauce

18 small slices of pepperoni
1 finely chopped green pepper
1 cup shredded Italian four-cheese blend

Instructions

Preheat oven to 400°F. Remove stem from portobello mushrooms and scrape out inside gills with a spoon and rinse well. Brush 1 1/2 tablespoon of olive oil all over mushrooms. Place on a large, rimmed non-stick baking sheet, hollow side up. Bake for 10 minutes and remove from oven. (Leave oven on.) Using paper towels, blot excess moisture from mushroom cavities and season with salt and pepper. Spread 1 tablespoon of jarred marinara tomato sauce in cavity of each mushroom. Divide 3 small slices of pepperoni and a little chopped green pepper, evenly among mushroom caps. Top each with 1/4 cup shredded Italian four-cheese blend. Return mushrooms to oven and bake until cheese is bubbling, about 10 minutes. Serve hot.

6 servings.

Gluten Free. Low Carb. Keto.

KETO PAN PIZZA

This is a true pan pizza and a true keto meal that loses the high-carb crust but gains high-praise pizza points for a fast food fix, no matter how you slice it.

Ingredients

1 3/4 cup shredded mozzarella cheese
1/4 cup grated Parmesan cheese
1/3 cup sliced pepperoni
1/3 cup chopped green pepper
1/3 cup sliced mushrooms
1/4 teaspoon dried oregano

Instructions

Evenly sprinkle the mozzarella cheese in a 10-inch non-stick pan in a thin layer to cover the bottom of the pan. Sprinkle evenly with Parmesan cheese. Place pan on burner and heat over medium heat. When the cheese starts to melt and bubble, top with pepperoni, bell peppers, mushrooms, and sprinkle with oregano. Continue cooking the pizza over medium heat until the bottom and edges are browned, about 8-10 minutes or until cheese is golden crisp. Remove the pan from the heat. Allow the pizza to cool and crisp up a bit, about 60 seconds, then use a flexible rubber spatula and carefully slide it around the edge of the pan pizza and onto a cutting board. With a round pizza cutter, cut the pan pizza into 8 small slices. Briefly place the pizza slices on paper towels to soak up extra grease, then serve.

2 servings.

Gluten Free. Low Carb. Keto.

NO-CARB CHICKEN CRUST PIZZA

Don't be a "chicken," try this surprisingly good option for a pizza with a high-protein, no-carb crust, using ground chicken.

Ingredients

Chicken Crust

1 lb ground chicken
2 cups shredded mozzarella cheese, (reserve 1 cup for after baking)
1/3 cup of Parmesan cheese

1 egg
1 teaspoon garlic powder
1 tsp dried oregano

Toppings

1 cup marinara sauce
1/2 cup mozzarella cheese

Any chopped veggie or meat pizza toppings you prefer

Instructions

Preheat oven to 400°F. Line pizza pan with parchment paper. Combine the chicken crust ingredients in a large mixing bowl. Form into a big ball. Place chicken ball on parchment paper-lined pizza pan. Cover with another sheet of parchment paper and roll out with rolling pin (or wine bottle or side of drinking glass) and pat with fingers, forming into a 1/2 inch thick circle. Slowly remove top parchment paper. Bake chicken crust in oven for 20-25 minutes or until top is browned. Remove from oven and carefully drain any accumulated grease. Spread the marinara sauce evenly over the cooked chicken crust mixture. Sprinkle half of the remaining mozzarella over the crust, then layer pizza toppings. Sprinkle the rest of the mozzarella cheese over the top. Bake in oven for an additional 10-20 minutes until cheese is slightly brown. Let cool for 5-10 minutes before slicing into the chicken crust pizza to serve.

4 servings.

Gluten Free. Low Carb. Keto.

FATHEAD PIZZA

For a classic copycat crust without the carbs, this fathead pizza recipe, as it's known, with the high-fat keto diet, comes together fast and gets raves reviews from the low-carb crowd, as long as you don't get offended by the name.

Ingredients

1 1/2 cups shredded mozzarella cheese
3/4 cup almond flour
2 Tbsp cream cheese
1 egg
Pinch of salt, to taste

1/2 tsp dried oregano
1/2 tsp garlic powder
1 cup marinara sauce
Any chopped veggie or meat pizza toppings you prefer

Instructions

Mix the shredded cheese and almond flour in a microwaveable bowl. Add the cream cheese. Microwave on HIGH for 1 minute. Stir, then microwave on high for another 30 seconds. Add the egg, salt, oregano, and any other spices, mix gently. Place in between 2 pieces of parchment paper and roll out with rolling pin (or wine bottle or side of drinking glass) into a circular pizza shape. Remove the top parchment paper slowly. If the mixture hardens and becomes difficult to work with, pop it back in the microwave for 10-20 seconds to soften again but not too long or you will cook the egg. With a fork, poke holes all over the pizza base to ensure it cooks evenly. Slide the parchment paper with the pizza base onto a baking sheet or pizza pan, and bake at 425°F for 12-15 minutes, or until brown. To make the base really crispy and sturdy, flip the pizza over (onto parchment paper) once the top has browned. Once cooked, remove from the oven, and add the marinara sauce and all the toppings you like. Make sure any meat is already cooked, as this time it goes back into the oven just to heat up the toppings and melt the cheese. Bake again at 425°F for 5 minutes.

4 servings.

Gluten Free. Low Carb. Keto.

FATHEAD PIZZA ROLLS

Once you are on a roll with the fathead pizza recipe, give this tasty twist a try. I know, I am so "punny and cheesy."

Ingredients

1 1/2 cups shredded mozzarella cheese
3/4 cup almond flour
2 Tbsp cream cheese
1 egg
Pinch of salt, to taste

1/2 tsp dried oregano
1/2 tsp garlic powder
1 cup marinara sauce
Any chopped veggie or meat pizza toppings you prefer

Instructions

Preheat oven to 400°F. Cover baking sheet with parchment paper. Sprinkle garlic salt and a small amount of almond flour on the surface of the paper. Melt the mozzarella and cream cheese in the microwave for 60 seconds. Stir almond flour and egg in with the melted cheese mixture to form the dough. Flatten the dough into a rectangular shape on the parchment paper-lined pan. Bake the dough for 3 minutes at 400°F. Remove from oven and lift edges of dough from parchment paper. Spread marinara sauce across the surface of the crust. Evenly distribute the rest of the pizza toppings over the sauce. Starting with one edge of the crust, gently roll into a log. Using a sharp knife, cut into slices. Lay slices flat on top of parchment paper-covered cookie sheet. Bake for 10-15 minutes, until dough becomes golden.

4 servings.

Gluten Free. Low Carb. Keto.

PEPPERONI PIZZA STUFFED CHICKEN

A simple way to "stuff" the family on a busy weeknight, full of protein and pizza flavour!

Ingredients

4 chicken breasts
2 tsp avocado oil
1 tsp garlic powder
1/2 tsp Italian seasoning
1/2 tsp salt

2 cups grated mozzarella, divided
1/4 cup Parmesan cheese
16 small slices pepperoni
1 cup marinara sauce
2-3 Fresh basil leaves

Instructions

Preheat oven to 375°F. Spray a 9x13 baking dish with non-stick spray or line with parchment paper. Place the chicken breasts on a cutting board. Use a sharp knife to cut a pocket into the side of each chicken breast. Drizzle both sides of the chicken with oil and season with the garlic powder, Italian seasoning, and salt. Place 1/4 cup of mozzarella in the pocket of each chicken breast. Add 2 slices of pepperoni over the cheese. Place the chicken in the prepared baking dish and drizzle with the pizza sauce. Spread the sauce out to cover the tops of the chicken. Sprinkle with the remaining mozzarella. Top with the Parmesan and remaining pepperoni slices. Bake, uncovered, for 30-35 minutes or until the chicken is cooked through and cheese begins to brown. Sprinkle with torn, fresh basil leaves before serving.

4 servings.

Gluten Free. Low Carb. Keto.

CHEESY CAULIFLOWER GARLIC FINGERS

For when you want extra veggies and less carbs in your crust, the power of cauliflower crust garlic fingers does the trick for this cheesy copy of a classic crowd-pleaser.

Ingredients

- 4 cups riced cauliflower, or about 1 large head of cauliflower
- 4 eggs
- 2 cups shredded mozzarella cheese
- 3 tsp oregano
- 4 cloves garlic, minced
- Salt and pepper, to taste
- 1 cup mozzarella cheese or more, for topping
- 1 cup of marinara sauce for dipping

Instructions

Preheat oven to 425°F. Line a large baking sheet with parchment paper. Make sure your cauliflower is roughly chopped in florets. Add the florets to your food processor or high-speed blender and pulse until cauliflower resembles rice. Place the cauliflower in a microwavable container and cover with lid. Microwave for 10 minutes. Let the cauliflower cool just until there's no more steam coming from it. Wrap the cauliflower in a dish towel, place over a sink or bowl, and squeeze out as much water as you can from it. Place the microwaved cauliflower in a large bowl and add the eggs, 2 cups of mozzarella, oregano, garlic, salt, and pepper. Mix everything together. Place mixture onto the prepared baking sheet and shape into either a round pizza shape or a rectangle for the garlic fingers. Bake the crust (no toppings yet) for about 25 minutes or until golden. Once golden, sprinkle with remaining mozzarella cheese and put back in the oven for another 5 minutes or until cheese has melted and browned. Slice into small rectangle-shape breadsticks and use marinara sauce for dipping if desired.

4 servings.

Gluten Free. Low Carb. Keto.

THE BEST WAY TO WARM UP LEFTOVER PIZZA

I couldn't provide you with all these ways to whip up healthier pizza at home without sharing with you the best way to warm up leftover pizza. This is also important for those times when you do take the night off from your easy eating kitchen and dial-in for take-out pizza.

But before we get to that, the best leftover pizza starts with how you, "leave it-over" or how you store it the night before.

I learned that the best way to store leftover pizza is, what I termed, the

Pizza P3 Method. Yes, I take my pizza making, cooking, eating, and storing-to-eat-again seriously! Line a **P**late or Tupperware container with **P**aper towels, then put on a layer of sliced **P**izza, then cover again with paper towels. Plate. Paper towel. Pizza. Paper towel. Pizza. Paper towel. Pizza. Repeat. (Provided you have that much pizza leftover, which would be rare in my household.) Then wrap the whole thing in plastic wrap. This will ensure ultimate freshness and flavour.

Reheat like a Rockstar

Don't you touch that microwave to reheat your "za!" Although that method may seem as easy eating as you can get, it results in a wet and rubbery slice of pizza that can only pass as a novelty chew toy for a dog. Pizza deserves better and so do you. Other tried methods like warming on a grill or in the oven, although slightly better than the microwave, take longer and still don't give you that original taste and texture that you crave.

The Pan is the Plan

Place a skillet on the stovetop burner and let it preheat over medium heat for 3-5 minutes. Place the pizza slice or slices, crust side down, flat in the pan and cover it with a lid—this is a crucial step. Without covering it, you risk the toppings and cheese not warming up enough. Let the pizza warm for 6-8 minutes, until the crust gets slightly crispy again and the cheese is warm and bubbly. Remove and enjoy the pleasure of pizza all over again!

SNACKS, SIDES AND SAUCES

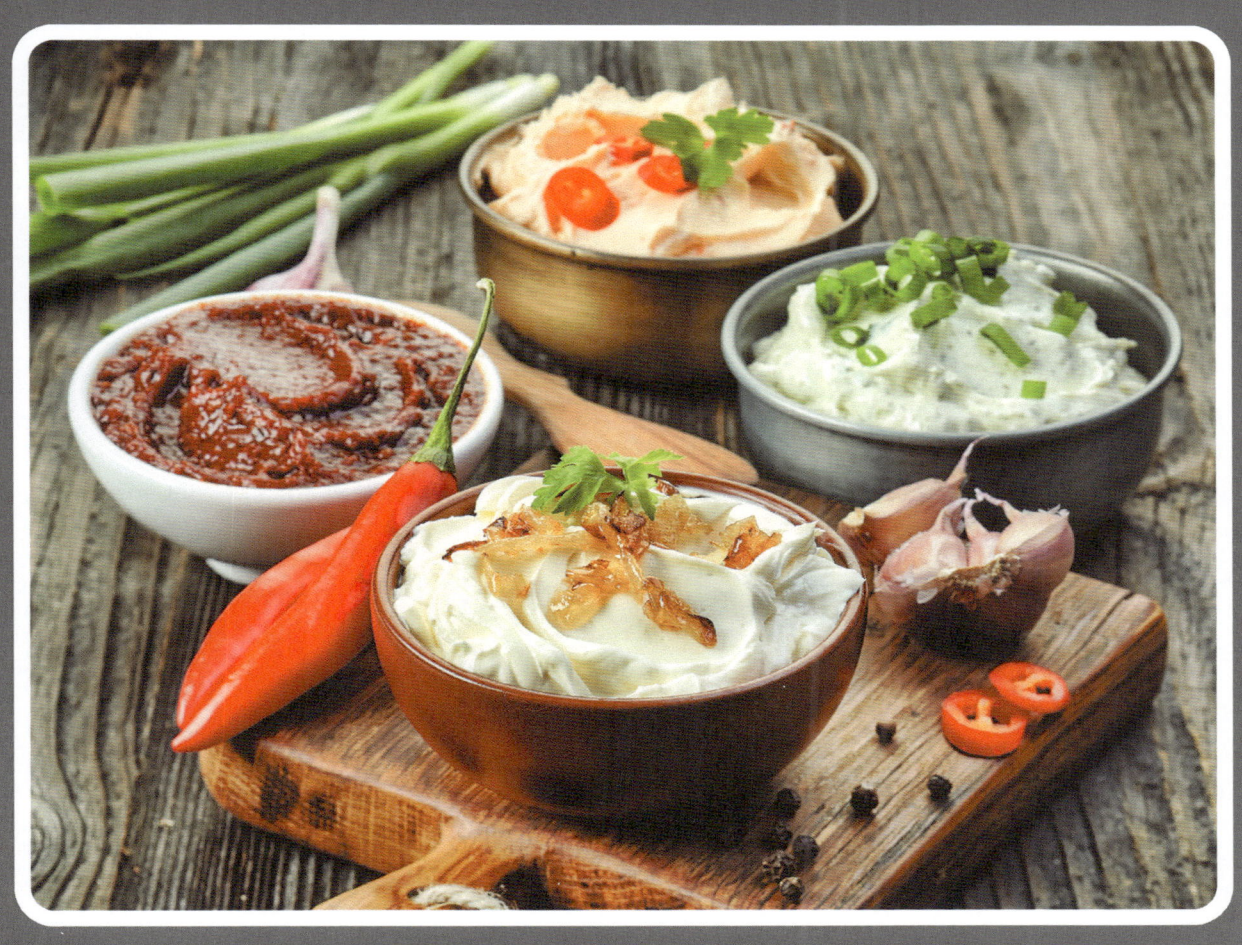

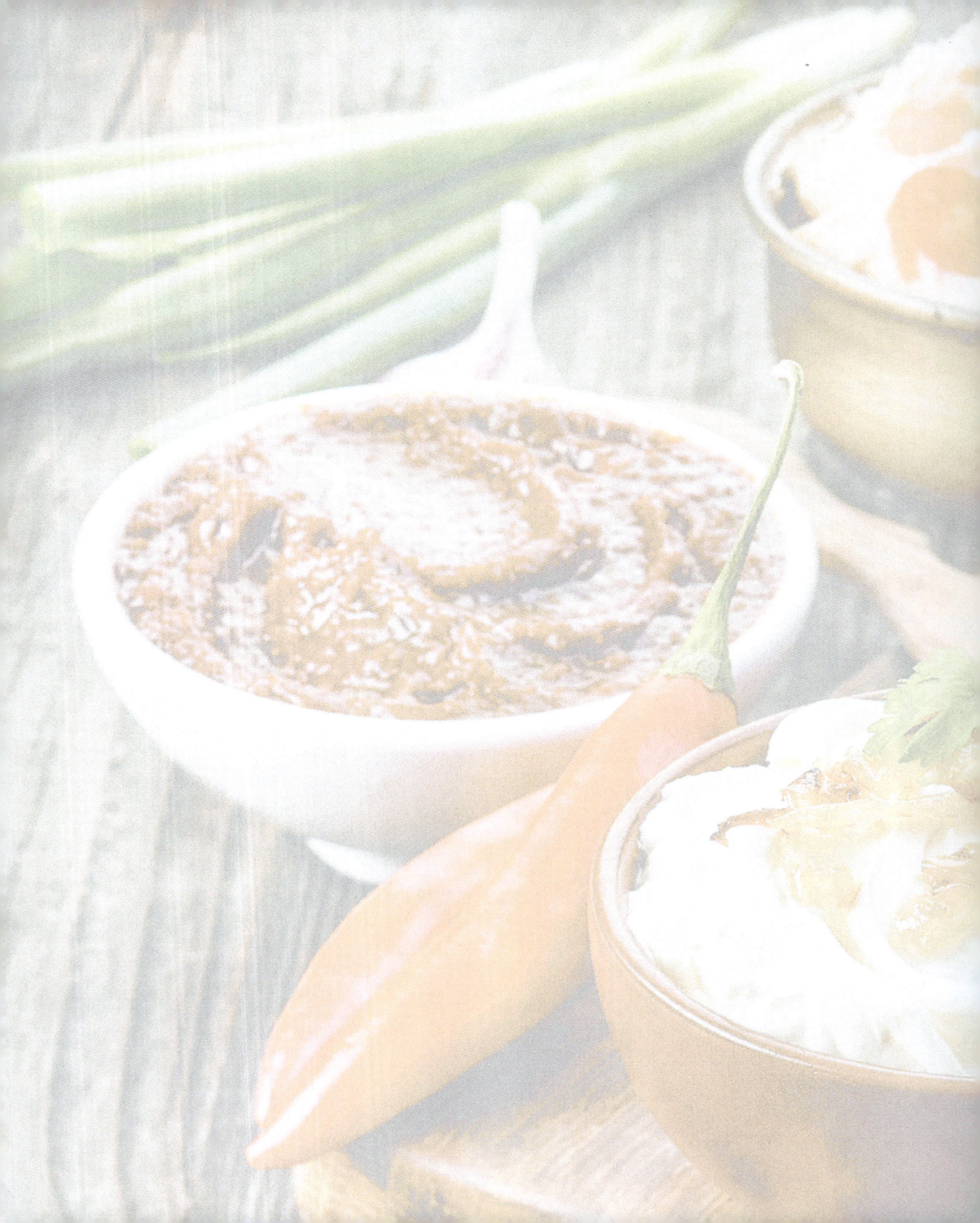

CHEESY BAKED ASPARAGUS

Such an easy cheesy way to serve up a side of veggies that will have your dinner guests "stalking" you for more.

Ingredients

1 lb of asparagus, stalks trimmed
2 Tbsp extra-virgin olive oil
3 cloves garlic
Juice of 1/2 lemon
1/2 tsp dried oregano

Red pepper flakes, for garnish
Kosher salt, to taste
2 cups of shredded mozzarella
Grated Parmesan, for garnish

Instructions

Preheat oven to 400°F. Cut off the bottom quarter of all the asparagus stems or snap them off where they will naturally break. In a large bowl, toss together asparagus, olive oil, garlic, lemon juice, and oregano. Season with salt and red pepper flakes. Lay out asparagus on a parchment paper-lined baking sheet then sprinkle with mozzarella. Bake in oven until tender for 15-20 minutes. Garnish with more red pepper flakes and Parmesan.

4 servings.

Gluten Free. Low Carb. Keto.

FRESH BASIL PESTO

You will go "nuts" for the fresh flavour that this pesto brings to many meals (like our Italian Goat Cheese Omelette).

Ingredients

2 cups fresh basil leaves, packed (you can sub half the basil leaves with baby spinach)
1/2 cup Romano or Parmesan cheese
1/2 cup extra-virgin olive oil

1/3 cup pine nuts or chopped walnuts
3 garlic cloves, minced
1/4 tsp salt, to taste
1/8 tsp black pepper, to taste

Instructions

Place the basil leaves and pine nuts or walnuts into the bowl of a food processor and pulse several times. Add the garlic and cheese and pulse several times more. Scrape down the sides of the food processor with a rubber spatula. While the food processor is running, slowly add the olive oil in a steady small stream. Adding the olive oil slowly, while the processor is running, will help it emulsify and help keep the olive oil from separating. Occasionally stop to scrape down the sides of the food processor. Stir in salt and pepper, add more to taste. Use this pesto in our goat cheese omelette recipe, toss with pasta for a quick sauce, dollop over baked potatoes, or spread onto crackers or toasted slices of bread.

*Basil pesto darkens when exposed to air, so to store, cover tightly with plastic wrap, making sure the plastic is touching the top of the pesto and not allowing the pesto to have contact with air. The pesto will stay greener longer that way.

Yields 1 cup.

Gluten Free. Low Carb. Keto.

LOW CARB CILANTRO LIME CAULIFLOWER RICE

Ingredients

1 large cauliflower, chopped into florets or 1 small bag of ready-made riced cauliflower
1 Tbsp extra-virgin olive oil
1 onion, chopped
2 scallions, sliced finely
2 garlic cloves
1/8 cup lime juice
1/4 cup fresh, chopped cilantro
Salt and pepper, to taste

Instructions

In a blender or food processor add 1 cup of cauliflower florets (one batch) and pulse quickly about 3-5 times or until the cauliflower is the same consistency of rice. Transfer to a large bowl and repeat with the next 1-cup batch of cauliflower florets until none remain. Heat a large non-stick pan over medium heat. Add olive oil, onions, scallions, and garlic and sauté for about 3 minutes on low-medium heat until soft and fragrant. Add the cauliflower "rice" and season with salt and pepper, to your taste. Increase burner temperature to high heat. Add the lime juice and cilantro. Stir mixture and cook while stirring frequently for about 6 minutes, or until the cauliflower is tender-crisp (soft on the inside, crispy on the outside).

4 servings.

*This goes great with Cilantro Lime Charred Chicken Thighs!

Gluten Free. Low Carb. Keto.

CRISPY BAKED FRENCH FRIES

Ingredients

4 large russet potatoes
3 Tbsp olive oil
1 Tbsp sea salt
1 tsp black pepper
1 tsp of paprika
1 tsp of garlic powder
1 tsp of dried oregano
1/2 cup grated Parmesan cheese

Instructions

Preheat oven to 425°F. Wash potatoes, leaving skin on (you can peel them if you prefer). Cut potatoes into desired size fries. Let potatoes soak in cold water in a bowl for at least 30 minutes if you have time. (This removes a lot of the starch to get crisper fries.) Remove from water and dry very well with paper towel or salad spinner. Toss with oil and seasonings in a big bowl or resealable bag. On a parchment paper-lined baking sheet, spread apart fries and bake for 15 minutes, turn fries over gently with spatula, and bake for additional 15 minutes or until golden brown. Remove from oven and sprinkle with Parmesan cheese while hot.

4 servings.

Gluten Free. Smart Carb.

FIT AND FAST FLAXSEED WRAP

"That's a wrap!" is what you will say for this leaner lunch option for a gluten-free wrap that comes together in just 2 minutes in the microwave. Then roll the wrap along with the cooking credits for you producing it.

Ingredients

3 Tbsp ground flax seed meal
1/4 tsp baking powder
1/4 tsp garlic powder
1/4 tsp paprika
1 pinch sea salt

1 Tbsp avocado oil or coconut oil (plus a little more to grease plate)
1 Tbsp water
1 egg

Instructions

Mix the ground flax seeds, baking powder, garlic powder, paprika, and salt in a bowl. Stir in avocado or melted coconut oil. Whisk in the egg and water until blended. Grease a microwave-safe dinner plate with the oil. Pour in the batter and tilt around plate to spread evenly. Microwave 2 minutes on high, until cooked. Wrap will be hot to touch so let stand five minutes. It should slide right off the plate but use a thin rubber spatula worked around the edges of the wrap to remove it, if needed. Flip and top with ingredients.

1 serving.

Gluten Free. Low Carb. Keto.

BUFFALO BAKED CHICKEN CHEESE DIP

Our most rave reviewed and go-to party dip for a crowd that's easy making and easier eating, with the classic taste, tang, and texture to create a party in your mouth all night long.

Ingredients

1 pkg (8 oz) cream cheese, softened
2 cups chopped, rotisserie chicken
1/2 cup mayo or sour cream
1 cup shredded mozzarella or cheddar cheese, divided
1/2 cup red hot sauce

Instructions

Mix softened cream cheese, chicken, mayo, hot sauce, and 1/2 cup of the shredded cheese together and shape into a big ball in a baking dish. Sprinkle remaining shredded cheese on top. Bake in a preheated oven on 350°F for 10-15 minutes. Broil on high the last 3-5 minutes until cheese begins to bubble and brown on top.

4-6 servings

*Choose sliced, cool cucumber or sliced, crispy bell peppers to go low-carb and cool down the spicy flavour, or use gluten-free crackers if desired.

6-8 servings.

Gluten Free. Low Carb. Keto

HEALTHY HOMEMADE TACO SEASONING

It's time to toss the taco mystery packets of seasoning stuffed in your taco kit, that is also stuffed with MSG, maltodextrin, additives, and processed oils, and make your own simple seasoning in minutes.

Ingredients

1 Tbsp chili powder
1/4 tsp garlic powder
1/4 tsp onion powder
1/4 tsp crushed red pepper flakes
1/4 tsp dried oregano

1/2 tsp paprika
1 1/2 tsp ground cumin
1 tsp sea salt
1 tsp black pepper

In a small bowl, mix together chili powder, garlic powder, onion powder, red pepper flakes, oregano, paprika, cumin, salt, and pepper. Store in an airtight container.

Yields 10 servings.

Gluten Free. Low Carb. Keto.

KUNG PAO BRUSSELS SPROUTS

Time to bring the WOW and POW to boring Brussels sprouts, with the salty, sweet and spicy Chinese combo of Kung Pao!

Ingredients

2 lb brussels sprouts, halved
2 Tbsp extra-virgin olive oil
Kosher salt
Freshly ground black pepper
1 Tbsp sesame oil
2 cloves garlic, minced
1 Tbsp cornstarch
1/2 cup low-sodium soy sauce (gluten free if preferred)
1/2 cup water
2 tsp apple cider vinegar
1 Tbsp hoisin sauce
1 Tbsp packed brown sugar
2 tsp sriracha sauce
Pinch crushed red pepper flakes
Sesame seeds, for garnish
Green onions, thinly sliced, for garnish
Chopped roasted peanuts, for garnish

Instructions

Preheat oven to 425°F. On a large, rimmed baking sheet lined with parchment paper, toss brussels sprouts with olive oil and season with salt and pepper. Bake until brussels sprouts are tender and slightly crispy, about 20 minutes. Transfer brussels sprouts to a large bowl (but keep the baking sheet close by). Preheat broiler. In a small skillet over medium heat, heat sesame oil. Add garlic and cook, until fragrant, about 1 minute. Stir in cornstarch. Add soy sauce, water, apple cider vinegar, hoisin sauce, brown sugar, and sriracha sauce.

Season with salt, pepper, and red pepper flakes.

Bring mixture to a boil, then reduce heat and simmer until thickened, about 3 minutes. Pour sauce over brussels sprouts and toss to combine. Return brussels sprouts to baking sheet and broil until brussels sprouts are glazed and sticky. Garnish with peanuts, sesame seeds, and green onions before serving.

4 servings.

Gluten Free. Low Carb.

SKINNY ZUCCHINI SKINS

Ditch loading up on the carbs from pub-style potato skins and go skinny with zucchini.

Ingredients

1/2 lb bacon
4 large zucchini
2 Tbsp extra-virgin olive oil
1/2 tsp chili powder
1/4 tsp ground cumin

Kosher salt
Freshly ground black pepper
2 cups shredded cheddar
1 cup sour cream, for garnish
2 green onions, thinly sliced, for garnish

Instructions

Preheat oven to 400°F. Cook bacon until crispy, about 8 to 10 minutes, then transfer to a paper towel-lined plate to drain and chop into small pieces. Cut zucchinis in half lengthwise. Using a large metal spoon, scoop out seeds from the insides, then cut each half crosswise into two pieces. Transfer zucchini to a large baking sheet and toss with olive oil. Season with chili powder, cumin, salt, and pepper. Bake until slightly tender, about 5 minutes. Top each piece of zucchini with cheese and bacon. Return to oven and bake until cheese is bubbly and zucchini is tender, about 10 minutes more. Garnish with sour cream and green onions before serving.

4-6 servings.

Gluten Free. Low Carb. Keto.

GARLIC PARMESAN KALE CHIPS

When you want to crush a chip craving fast, keep the satisfying salt, spice, and crunch but leave the carbs and calories. Feel good about going green to stay lean, with kale chips. Betcha can't eat just one!

Ingredients

1 medium-sized bunch of kale
2 tsp extra-virgin olive oil
1 tsp of sea salt
1/2 tsp of garlic powder
1 Tbsp of grated Parmesan cheese

Instructions

Preheat your oven to 350°F. Line a large baking sheet with parchment paper. Tear the kale leaves off the stems and away from the chewy veins of the kale and into chip-sized pieces. Wash and dry kale, making sure the leaves are completely dry by using a salad spinner or drying with a paper towel. If there's any moisture left on the leaves, you'll end up with soggy kale chips.

Arrange the pieces of kale on the baking sheet, being sure to not overcrowd the pan with leaves, keeping them spread apart, as overlapped leaves will steam and come out soggy not crisp. With larger bunches of kale, it's best to use two pans.

Drizzle the olive oil as evenly over the kale as possible. Using your hands, gently massage the oil into the kale leaves, making sure to massage the oil well into all the folds and onto the entire surface of each of the kale leaves. Once you've finished massaging the kale, evenly sprinkle the sea salt, garlic powder, and Parmesan over the kale and add the pan to your preheated oven. Bake for 15 minutes, but watch the pan closely for the last 5 minutes to prevent over-browning and burning. You want a nice balance between crispiness and chewiness without any burnt edges. Remove the pan from the oven and leave the kale chips on the pan for 3-5 minutes before serving so they can crisp up even more.

2-4 servings.

Gluten Free. Low Carb. Keto

THE BEST BAKED BROCCOLI

This superfood will create super fans of all ages in your household once they bite into this fit and flavourful baked broccoli.

Ingredients

2 lbs frozen broccoli florets, or fresh cut florets
3-4 tablespoons extra-virgin olive oil
Juice from half a lemon
1 Tbsp sea salt

2-3 garlic cloves, minced or 1 Tbsp of garlic powder
Freshly ground black pepper
1/4 cup grated Parmesan cheese, or to taste

Instructions

Preheat oven to 425°F. In a large bowl, toss the broccoli florets and minced garlic with olive oil and lemon juice until lightly coated. Sprinkle salt over the broccoli and toss to coat. Arrange the broccoli florets in a single layer on a large baking sheet that has been rubbed with some olive oil or lined with parchment paper. Roast for 20-30 minutes in the oven until cooked through (check by poking with a fork, should be fork-tender) and lightly browned. The browned bits are the best, so don't worry if you see some charring. Put the roasted broccoli back in the bowl and toss with lots of freshly ground black pepper and the grated Parmesan cheese. Be generous with the black pepper, broccoli loves it!

4 servings.

Gluten Free. Low Carb. Keto

PIZZA POPCORN

Movie night and pizza night, "is in the bag"! With this tasty twist on popcorn.

Ingredients

1 1/4 cup unpopped corn kernels
3 Tbsp coconut oil
1/2 cup butter
1 teaspoon paprika
1 1/2 teaspoon garlic powder
1/2 teaspoon sea salt

1/2 teaspoon dried oregano
1/2 teaspoon dried basil
Dash of hot sauce (optional)
1 1/2 cups freshly grated Parmesan cheese
Pinch or two of paprika for garnish

Instructions

Pop your kernels, the natural, easy eating way! Set a burner to medium-high heat. Add coconut oil to a large pot with a lid. Add the corn kernels and cover the pot. When you hear the first sound of kernels popping, reduce heat to medium-low and allow the kernels to pop completely. Every minute or so, give the pot a shake to ensure all your kernels have popped. Remove from heat and set aside. You can also choose to pop popcorn kernels using a popcorn maker or microwave in a closed brown paper bag.

Make the pizza sauce mixture: Preheat your oven to 350°F. Melt the butter in a small skillet or saucepan over medium heat. When the butter has melted, add the paprika, garlic powder, salt, oregano, basil, and hot sauce and stir to combine. Drizzle the butter mixture over the popped popcorn, tossing to ensure all the popcorn is well coated. Add the Parmesan cheese and toss well. Pour the popcorn mixture onto a large baking sheet and roast for 10-15 minutes, stirring once after about 8 minutes. Sprinkle with an additional pinch or two of paprika and some fresh parsley and serve immediately!

4 servings.

Gluten Free. Smart carb.

SALSA GUACAMOLE

Combining these two-party players of salsa and avocado always brings you a winning dip come game time.

Ingredients

3 avocados
1 1/2 tsp lime juice
2 Tbsp salsa
1 tsp garlic powder

1 tsp cumin
Salt, to taste
Optional: chopped cilantro, hot sauce.

Instructions

Using a sharp chef's knife, slice through one side of the avocado lengthwise until you feel the knife hit the pit. Rotate the avocado, keeping the knife steady, to make a cut all around the pit. Twist the two halves apart. To remove the pit, aim the bottom half of your knife blade at the pit and whack into it, using enough force that the knife sticks into the pit. Twist the knife to pull out the pit. Flick the pit off the knife with a push of your thumb or tap it off the side of a bowl. Then scoop out the flesh with a spoon or squeeze the flesh with your hand until the flesh slides out. Add the lime juice, salsa, cumin, and garlic powder. Mash it together with a fork until you get the consistency you prefer. Add a pinch of salt and taste. If you can't taste the avocado much, add a bit more salt and spices. Stir in cilantro and hot sauce at the end if desired.

4 servings

Gluten Free. Low Carb. Keto.

CHEESY ZUCCHINI SPINACH ARTICHOKE BITES

A tasty and healthy appetizer that is Popeye approved and that will have the eyes of your guests popping!

Ingredients

4 oz cream cheese, softened
2/3 cup shredded mozzarella
1/4 cup freshly grated Parmesan
1/2 cup canned artichoke hearts, drained and chopped
1/2 cup frozen spinach, thawed and drained

2 Tbsp sour cream
2 cloves garlic, minced
Pinch of crushed red pepper flakes
Salt and pepper, to taste
3 medium zucchini, cut into 1/2" rounds

Instructions

Preheat oven to 400°F and line a large baking sheet with parchment paper. In a medium bowl, combine cream cheese, mozzarella, Parmesan, artichokes, spinach, sour cream, garlic, and crushed red pepper. Season with salt and pepper. Spread a tablespoon of cream cheese mixture on top of each zucchini sliced round. Bake until zucchini is tender and cheese is melty, around 15 minutes. To brown the cheese mixture, broil on high for 2 to 3 minutes.

4 servings.

Gluten Free. Low Carb. Keto.

SOUPS AND SALADS

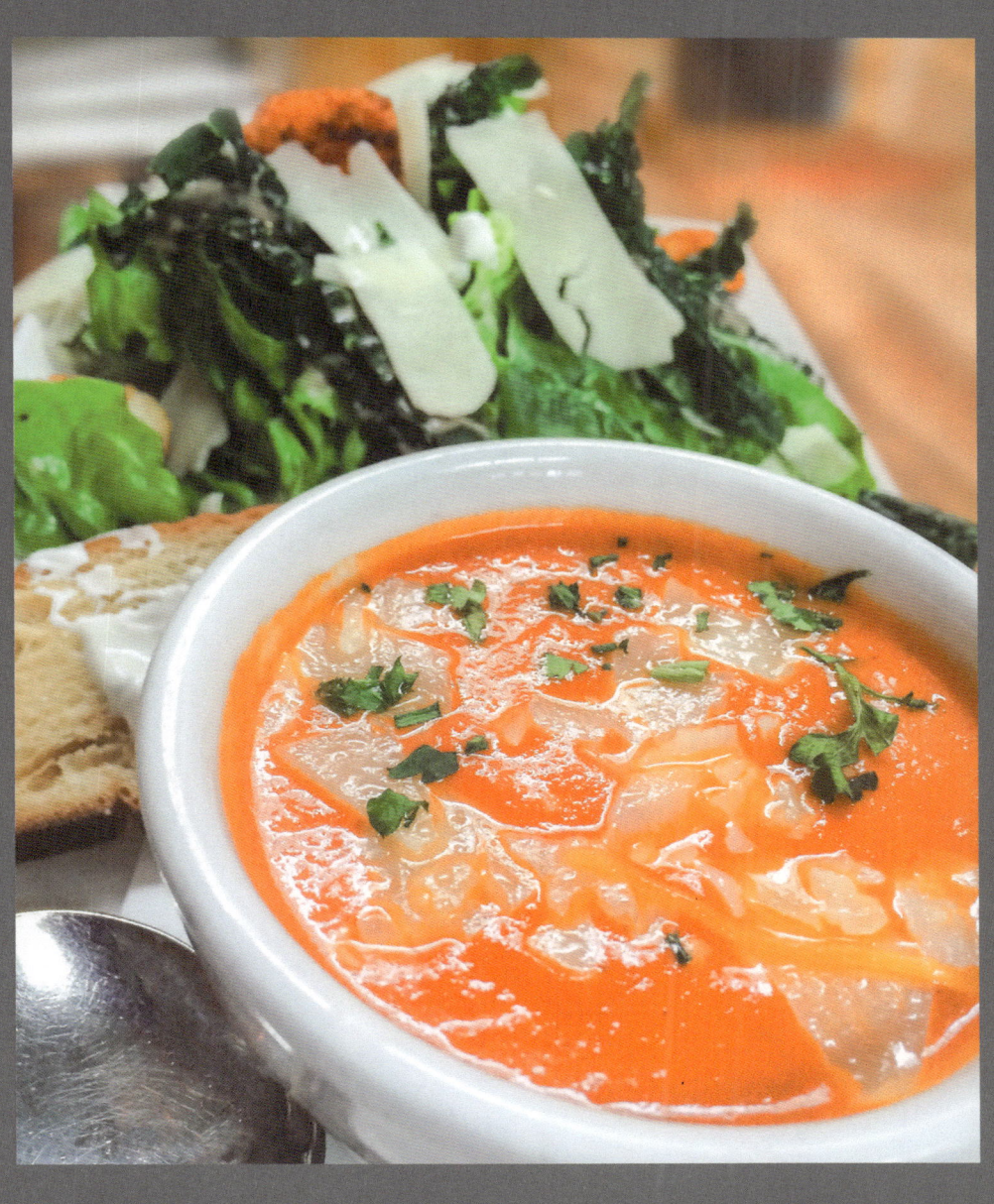

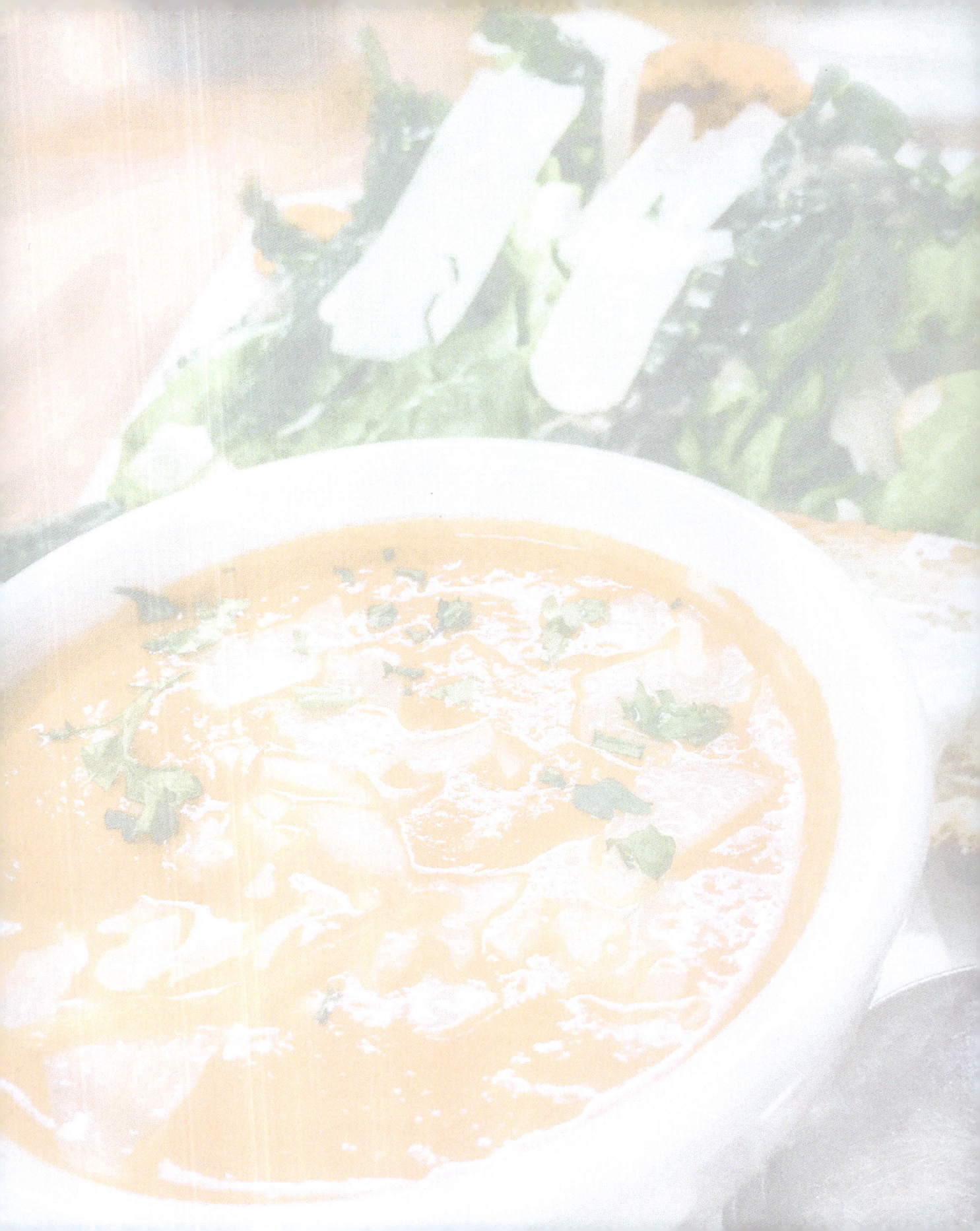

THREE-INGREDIENT TOMATO SOUP

This simple and surprising trio of ingredients, tomatoes, onion, and stock, "blends" together perfectly for when you want the classic comfort of a warm bowl of simmered and savoury tomato soup without the can.

Ingredients

4 Tbsp unsalted butter
1/2 large onion, cut into large wedges
1 (28-oz) can crushed tomatoes,

1 1/2 cups water, low sodium vegetable stock, or chicken stock
1/2 teaspoon sea salt, or more, to taste

Instructions

Melt butter over medium heat in a pot or large saucepan. Add onion wedges, water or stock, can of crushed tomatoes, and salt. Bring to a simmer. Cook uncovered for about 40 minutes. Stir occasionally and add additional salt as needed. Blend the soup in the pot using a handheld immersion blender or pour the soup into a regular blender. (Be careful it's hot!) If you use a regular blender, don't fill the blender all the way to the top as you usually would since the soup is hot, and puree in batches if needed. To allow the steam to escape and prevent the blender lid from popping off which can cause a hot mess, remove the centre insert of the lid and cover the hole loosely with a kitchen towel while blending on low until soup is semi-smooth. Top with freshly cracked black pepper and chopped fresh basil.

4 servings.

Gluten Free. Low Carb.

CREAMY CAULIFLOWER SOUP

Serve up this "soup-er" food soup that is heavy on flavour but will make you feel lighter.

Ingredients

1 large head cauliflower, cut into florets or 1 bag of frozen florets
1 large onion, sliced or chopped
4 cloves garlic, minced
Salt and pepper, to taste
2 Tbsp olive oil
5 cups chicken or vegetable broth
2 tsp fresh chopped parsley, thyme, or rosemary

1/2 cup heavy cream
2 Tbsp finely chopped chives or green onions
1/2 cup diced bacon pre-cooked (to serve)
1/4 cup shredded cheddar cheese, mozzarella or Parmesan

Instructions

Preheat the oven to 425°F. Line a large rimmed baking sheet with parchment paper. Combine cauliflower, onion, and garlic on the baking sheet. Season with a generous amount of salt and pepper. Toss with olive oil until evenly coated in oil. Arrange in a single layer. Bake for 15 minutes. Toss the cauliflower through the onions and garlic, then return to the oven and bake for a further 10-15 minutes until the cauliflower is caramelized on the edges and fork-tender. Transfer cauliflower to a pot. Add stock and herbs. Bring to a simmer over medium heat. Cook, stirring occasionally for 15 minutes to let the flavours blend. When cauliflower is soft, remove from the heat and let cool for 5 minutes.

Blend the soup in the pot using a handheld immersion blender or pour the soup into a regular blender. (Be careful it's hot!) If you use a regular blender, don't fill the blender all the way to the top as you usually would since the soup is hot, and puree in batches, if needed. To allow the steam to escape and prevent the blender lid from popping off which can cause a hot mess, remove the centre insert of the lid and cover the hole loosely with a kitchen towel while blending on low until soup is semi-smooth.

Add the cream and blend until smooth. To serve, top bowls of soup with chopped cooked bacon, shredded cheese, and chopped chives or green onion.

6 servings.

Gluten Free. Low Carb. Keto.

ITALIAN CHICKEN SOUP

Warm your soul and go back for another bowl, of this Italian chicken soup that is the best medicine meal to have when you are feeling under the weather.

Ingredients

2 Tbsp extra-virgin olive oil
1 medium onion, chopped
2 carrots, chopped
1 celery stalk, chopped
2 cloves garlic, minced
Kosher salt
Freshly ground black pepper

1 tsp of dried oregano
4 cups or 1 (32 fl oz. carton) of chicken stock
1 (32-oz) can diced tomatoes in juice
2 lbs cooked chicken breast or rotisserie chicken breast, chopped
Fresh basil leaves for garnish

Instructions

In a large, heavy pot, heat the oil over medium-high heat until hot. Stir in the onion, carrots, celery, 1/2 teaspoon salt, and 1/4 teaspoon pepper, and cook, stirring occasionally, until golden, about 6 minutes. Stir in the stock, tomatoes with their juices, and cooked chicken, then bring to a gentle boil. Simmer for 20 to 25 minutes. Season the soup with salt and pepper to taste, then serve.

6 servings.

Gluten Free. Low Carb.

EASY CHEESY BROCCOLI CHEDDAR SOUP

Real cheddar makes it better! Enjoy this creamy comfort in a bowl, with this Easy Cheesy Broccoli Cheddar Soup.

Ingredients

1/3 cup butter
1 yellow onion, chopped
4 cloves garlic, finely chopped
1/3 cup gluten-free flour blend
2 cups or (16 fl oz.) low-sodium chicken stock
3 cups half-and-half, or milk (any kind)
3/4 tsp salt, or more to taste
1/2 tsp black pepper, or more to taste

1 tsp vegetable stock powder (or chicken bouillon powder)
1 tsp mustard powder
1 tsp garlic powder
1 pound (450 grams) broccoli florets, cut into small pieces
2 large carrots, peeled and grated
2 cups full-fat old cheddar cheese, grated

Instructions

Melt the butter in a large pot over medium heat. Fry the onion until fragrant (about 2 minutes). Add in the garlic and cook for a further minute. Whisk in the flour and cook for a few minutes or until golden brown. Reduce heat to medium-low and slowly pour in the chicken stock and half-and-half, stirring well to combine and dissolve the flour into the liquid. Season with salt and pepper, stock powder, mustard powder and garlic powder. Give it a good mix and allow to cook and thicken for about 5 minutes, while stirring occasionally. Add in the broccoli and carrots and gently simmer for another 20 minutes, until broccoli is completely tender. Mix in cheddar cheese and stir until just combined. (It's important to use a full-fat cheddar cheese that you grate yourself. Don't use pre-grated cheese in ziptop bags because that cheese won't incorporate well and the flavour of the soup depends on it.) Add in extra salt and/or pepper to taste.

6 servings.

Gluten Free. Low Carb.

CLASSIC CHOPPED COBB SALAD

One late night in 1937, Bob Cobb, then owner of The Brown Derby restaurant in Hollywood, chopped and tossed together these ingredients left in his fridge and the comforting and creamy Cobb salad "star" was born, and it has been a fan favourite at restaurants, and at home, ever since.

Ingredients

1/3 cup red wine or balsamic vinegar
1 Tbsp Dijon mustard
2/3 cup extra-virgin olive oil
Salt and freshly ground black pepper
1 head romaine lettuce or salad greens mix, coarsely chopped
4 hard-boiled eggs, peeled and sliced
1 cup of cooked, chopped chicken breast
2 slices of cooked, chopped bacon or smoked ham
1 avocado, thinly sliced
4 oz crumbled blue cheese or goat cheese
1 cup cherry tomatoes, halved
2 Tbsp finely chopped green onion (optional)

Instructions

In a mason jar or shaker bottle, shake together vinegar, mustard, and oil, and season with salt and pepper. On a large platter, spread out lettuce or green salad mix, then add sliced hard-boiled eggs, chopped chicken, bacon or ham, avocado, blue or goat cheese, and cherry tomatoes. Season with salt and pepper, drizzle with dressing, and garnish with green onion if desired.

4 servings.

Gluten Free. Low Carb. Keto.

GREEK SUMMER SALAD

Taste the trip of a cool and crisp salty breeze on a warm summer day off the coast of the Mediterranean, with this go-to Greek summer salad.

Ingredients

1 cup grape or cherry tomatoes, halved
1 cucumber, thinly sliced into halves
1 cup halved Kalamata or sliced black olives
1/2 red onion, thinly sliced
3/4 cup crumbled feta cheese

2 Tbsp red wine vinegar
Juice of 1/2 a lemon
1 tsp dried oregano
Salt and freshly ground black pepper
1/4 cup extra-virgin olive oil

Instructions

In a large bowl, stir together tomatoes, cucumber, olives, and red onion. (If you find the taste of raw red onion too strong, soak the slices in cold water for 10 to 15 minutes, then drain and pat dry. This helps tame the spice.) Drop in the crumbled feta. In a small bowl, make dressing and drizzle dressing over salad.

Dressing

Combine vinegar, lemon juice, and oregano, and season with salt and pepper. Slowly add olive oil, whisking to combine.

2 servings.

Gluten Free. Low Carb. Keto.

FAST AND FLAVOURFUL FIVE-MINUTE ARUGULA SIDE SALAD

This arugula side salad with the perfect pairing of peppery arugula, Parmesan shavings, lemon and olive oil is so fast, fresh, and flavourful. It only calls for five easy eating ingredients and can be made in less than 5 minutes!

Ingredients

2 cups fresh, baby arugula
2 Tbsp freshly grated Parmesan cheese, plus extra shavings as garnish
2 tsp extra-virgin olive oil
2 tsp freshly squeezed lemon juice
1 tsp freshly cracked black pepper

Instructions

Add arugula and shaved Parmesan to a large mixing bowl. Drizzle evenly with olive oil and lemon juice, and sprinkle with black pepper. Toss until combined.

Serve immediately, garnished with extra Parmesan if desired.

2 servings.

Gluten Free. Low Carb. Keto.

CHUNKY CHOPPED CHICKEN SALAD

It's OK to call the chicken "chunky", it has tough skin! So mix up this fast and flavourful high protein low-carb lunch.

Ingredients

2 cups leftover chopped, cooked chicken breast or rotisserie chicken breast
1 scallion, finely diced
1/3 cup mayonnaise or plain Greek yogurt
1/2 red bell pepper, finely diced
1/3 cup diced celery
1 tsp Dijon mustard
1/2 tsp lemon juice or apple cider vinegar
1/2 tsp ground cumin
Salt and pepper, to taste

Instructions

Stir together mayonnaise or Greek yogurt, scallions, Dijon, lemon juice or apple cider vinegar, cumin, and salt and pepper. Toss with remaining ingredients. Serve on large lettuce leaves or salad greens for lower carb option than bread.

2 servings.

Gluten Free. Low Carb. Keto.

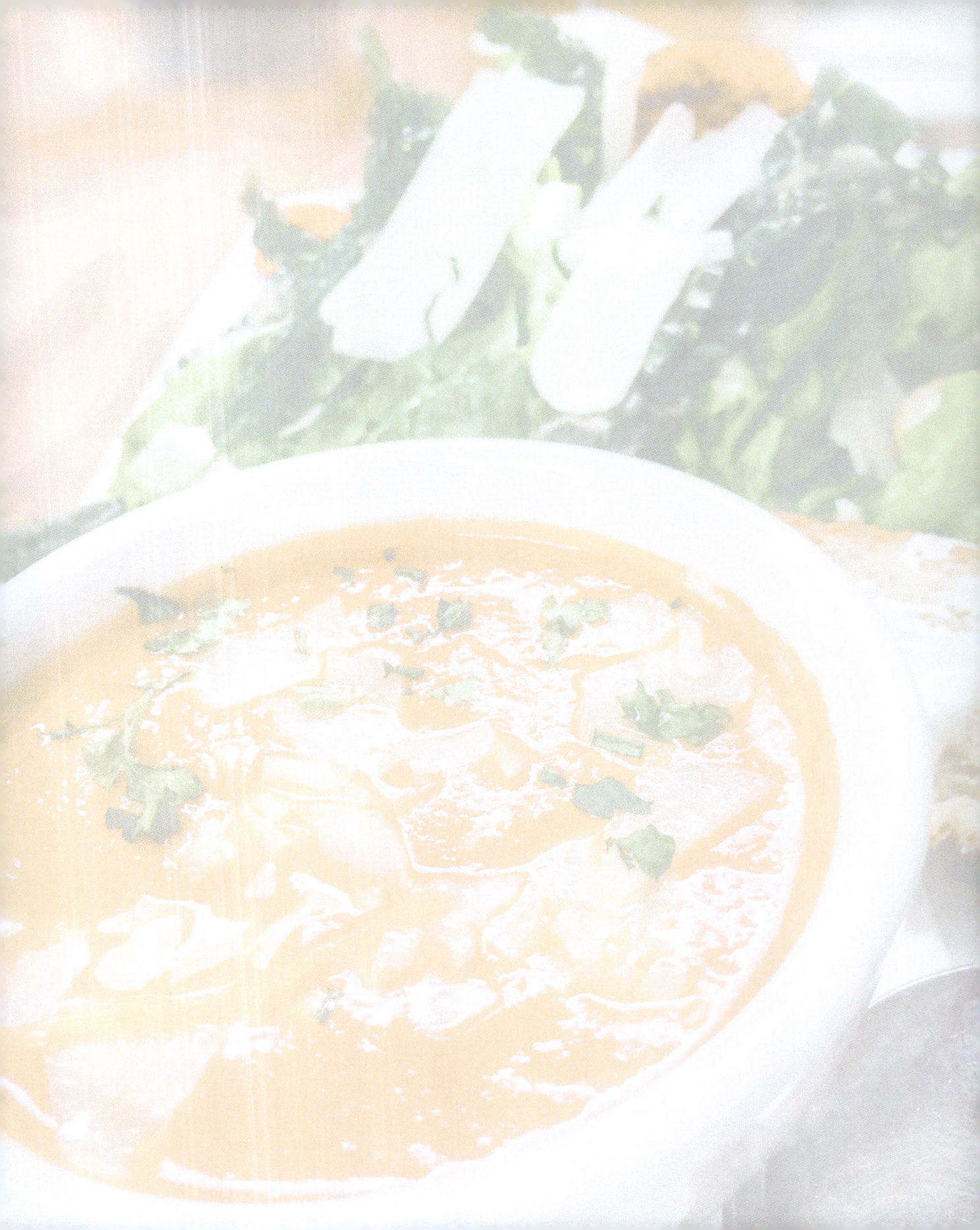

SWEET TREATS

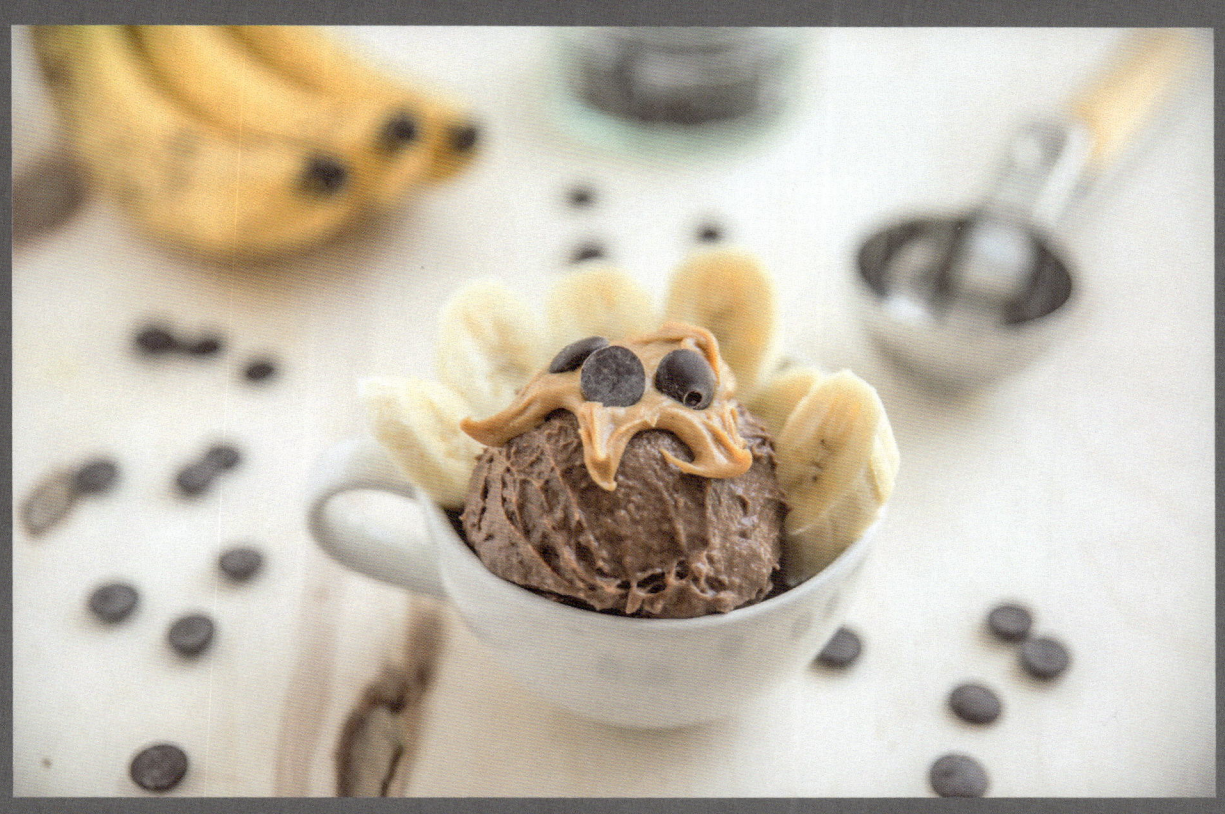

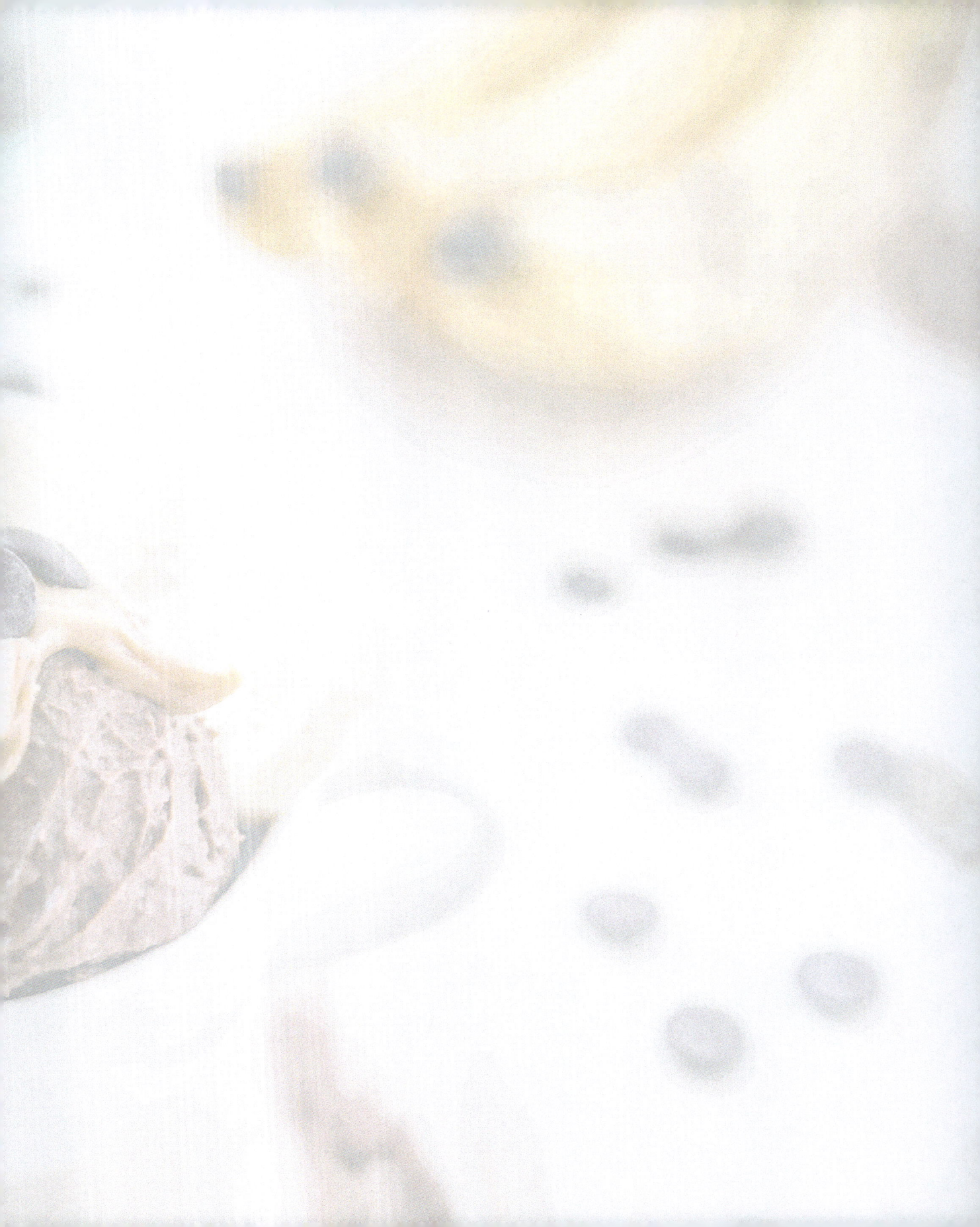

CHOCOLATE PEANUT BUTTER PROTEIN NICE-CREAM

Get instant ice cream with this healthy hack of ingredients that you probably already have in your kitchen. Kids love to make this, almost as much as they love to scream for this "nice"-cream!

Ingredients

4 frozen overripe bananas
1/4 cup natural peanut butter
1/3 cup cocoa powder
1 scoop chocolate whey or plant protein powder
1/4 tsp pure vanilla extract
1/8 tsp salt

Instructions

Make sure the bananas are at least partially brown before chopping and freezing them. Combine all ingredients in a high-power blender or food processor. Process until completely smooth, adding a little milk of choice if your blender isn't strong enough to handle the frozen banana. (If you're not using a high-speed blender and don't want to add any liquid, simply thaw the bananas a bit before blending.) Either serve immediately as soft serve or freeze for up to an hour before scooping out with an ice cream scoop.

4 servings.

Gluten Free. Smart Carb.

STRAWBERRY FROZEN YOGURT BARK

Break up your routine for a healthy snack or even breakfast, with this protein rich frozen yogurt bark that is sweet, salty and simple!

Ingredients

2 cups plain Greek yogurt
1/4 cup honey, plus 2 Tbsp
2 tsp vanilla extract
1/8 tsp fine salt

1/2 tsp cinnamon
1 cup diced strawberries
1/2 cup crushed walnuts

Instructions

Line a rimmed baking sheet with parchment paper (make sure it fits in your freezer, otherwise line two large plates instead). Set aside. Whisk the yogurt, 1/4 cup of the honey, vanilla, salt, and cinnamon together in a medium bowl. Pour onto the baking sheet and use a rubber spatula to spread into an even layer about 1/2-inch thick (it will not reach to the edges of the baking sheet). Place the strawberries, crushed walnuts, and remaining 2 tablespoons honey in a small bowl and mix gently to combine. Scatter the strawberry-nut mixture evenly over the yogurt. Freeze uncovered until solid, about 4 hours. Pick up the bark by grasping the parchment paper and lifting it up and onto a cutting board. Cut into serving pieces and serve immediately, or keep frozen in a resealable plastic bag.

8 servings.

Gluten Free. Smart Carb.

PROTEIN POPSICLES

Cool down and beat the heat on a hot summer's day by popping this sweet healthy treat out of the freezer and into to your mouth, lickety split!

Ingredients

1 cup unsweetened vanilla or chocolate almond milk
2 scoops of vanilla or chocolate whey or plant protein powder
1 banana or 1/3 cup plain Greek yogurt
1 Tbsp of honey
Pinch of salt
10 popsicle molds

Instructions

Place all the ingredients in a blender and blend until smooth. Prepare 10 popsicle molds. Fill each mold with the blended smoothie. Insert the popsicle sticks, and freeze for at least 6 hours to completely freeze the popsicles. Dip the popsicle mold in hot water for a few seconds (or under running hot water), to make it easier to remove them.

Yields 10 popsicles.

Gluten Free. Smart Carb.

*Pretty much all typical protein smoothie ingredients can work for protein popsicles. Try different protein powder flavours, different liquid base milks, like dairy, unsweetened nut milks, or even coconut water. You can combine liquid layers, like chocolate and vanilla frozen in one mold (by freezing one half at a time), or add some nut butter, and especially any frozen fruit like berries, pineapple or mango for a tropical taste.

PEANUT BUTTER PROTEIN CHOCOLATE COLD BREW COFFEE

Skip the fancy coffee shop line-up and save yourself some bucks by whipping up this healthy hack on cold brew coffee and you will be the real "star."

Ingredients

1 cup cold leftover coffee
1 scoop of chocolate whey or plant protein powder
1 Tbsp of peanut butter powder
4 ice cubes

1/3 cup unsweetened chocolate almond milk
2 drops liquid stevia natural sweetener
1/8 tsp cinnamon
1 square of 85% dark chocolate, finely chopped

Instructions

Place all ingredients (except the dark chocolate, cinnamon, and 2 ice cubes) in a blender. Blend on high until combined and creamy. Pour back into a large coffee cup, mug, or glass filled with 2 more ice cubes and top with a sprinkle of finely chopped, dark chocolate shavings and a sprinkle of cinnamon.

1 serving.

Gluten Free. Low Carb. Keto.

PEANUT BUTTER PROTEIN MUFFINS

Have a gourmet muffin with some protein power, that will help give you muscles instead of a muffin top.

Ingredients

Muffins

1 cup almond flour
1/2 cup coconut flour
2 Tbsp peanut butter powder
1 scoop of chocolate or vanilla whey or plant protein powder
1 1/2 tsp baking powder
1 tsp xantham gum

1/2 tsp salt
1/4 cup natural granulated sweetener
4 Tbsp applesauce
1 whole small banana, mashed
1/2 cup coconut milk
1 egg

Peanut Butter Glaze

3 Tbsp peanut butter powder

2 Tbsp water

Instructions

Mix together almond flour, coconut flour, peanut butter powder, protein powder, baking powder, xanthan gum, salt, and natural sweetener in a large bowl. Add the applesauce and mashed banana and stir together. Mix the coconut milk and egg together and then add it to the flour mixture and mix just until combined. Place the batter in a lined or well-greased muffin tin (about 3 Tbsp in each tin). Bake at 350°F for 10-14 minutes. Cool muffins for about 10 minutes. For the glaze, add the peanut butter powder and water and mix well. Dip muffin tops in the glaze or drizzle on top.

Yields 12 muffins.

*You can use melted peanut butter in place of peanut butter powder if needed.

Gluten Free. Smart Carb.

NO-BAKE PEANUT BUTTER PROTEIN BROWNIE BALLS

Rock and roll like a baller for a nutritious treat that is easy to make, no-bake, and with the classic combo of peanut butter and chocolate.

Ingredients

1 cup rolled oats (use gluten free if preferred)
1 scoop of chocolate whey or plant protein powder
1/2 cup natural peanut butter
1/2 cup low sugar mini chocolate chips
1/4 cup pure maple syrup
2 Tbsp cocoa powder
2 Tbsp chia seeds
1/4 tsp salt (optional)

Instructions

Place oats and peanut butter in a food processor. Pulse a few times until the oats are coarsely ground and just mixed with the peanut butter. Add chocolate chips, maple syrup, cocoa powder, protein powder, chia seeds, and (optional) salt. Pulse until well mixed. If the mixture seems too dry (the consistency will vary depending on the peanut butter used) pulse in more maple syrup, a tablespoon at a time, until the desired, slightly sticky, easy to roll, consistency is achieved. Using clean hands, grab a small amount of the mixture, press it together between your hands, and roll into a roughly 1-inch sized ball. Place the ball on a parchment-lined pan and repeat with remaining mixture.

Once finished, place pan in the freezer until balls are no longer sticky. Transfer balls to a freezer-safe container for storage. (You can store them in the fridge, but I like to store them in the freezer until I'm ready to enjoy a bite or two.) When ready to eat, let thaw (if frozen) for a minute or two before enjoying.

Yields 15-20 small brownie balls.

Gluten Free. Smart Carb.

PALEO PROTEIN BANANA BREAD

There's nothing like the aroma of fresh banana bread baking in the oven, but it's the taste and texture of this high-protein gluten-free banana bread that will drive you wild.

Ingredients

4 overripe bananas (2 1/2 cups mashed)
4 eggs
1/2 cup almond butter
4 Tbsp melted butter
1/2 cup almond flour
1 scoop of vanilla whey or plant protein powder

1 Tbsp cinnamon
1 Tbsp baking soda
1 Tbsp baking powder
1 tsp vanilla
Pinch of sea salt
1 Tbsp of crushed walnuts for topping

Instructions

Preheat your oven to 350°F. Combine your bananas, eggs, nut butter, and butter in a blender, food processor, or mixing bowl and mix well (if using a mixing bowl, you need a good hand-mixer). Once all of your ingredients are blended, add in your almond flour, protein powder, cinnamon, baking soda, baking powder, vanilla, and sea salt, and mix well. Pour your batter in a greased loaf or silicon pan and spread evenly. Top with crushed walnuts. Place in your preheated oven and bake for 55-60 minutes or until a toothpick inserted into the centre comes out clean. Remove from oven and flip bread out gently onto a cooling rack. Let cool to slice and serve.

Yields one loaf.

* If you want to make these into muffins, use the same recipe and pour batter into greased muffin tins and bake approximately for 30 minutes.

Gluten Free. Smart Carb.

CHOCOLATE CHUNKY MONKEY BARS

When you feel like monkeying around in the kitchen, these brownie-like bars bring together the creamy combination of peanut butter, banana, and chocolate.

Ingredients

2 large overripe bananas
1/2 cup crunchy peanut butter or almond butter
3 eggs
1/4 cup coconut oil melted
1 cup almond flour
3 Tbsp coconut flour

1/2 tsp baking soda
1/4 tsp salt
1/3 cup low sugar mini chocolate chips
1 oz 85% dark chocolate (optional topping)
1/2 Tbsp butter

Instructions

Preheat oven to 350°F. Grease a 9x13 baking pan with coconut oil (or use a non-stick silicone pan). Peel bananas and mash with a fork until mushy and smooth. Add eggs, coconut oil, almond butter, almond flour, coconut flour, baking soda, and salt. Mix thoroughly to form a batter. Fold in chocolate chips. Pour batter into prepared baking sheet, and spread batter out evenly with a spatula or spoon. Bake for 18-20 minutes. Let cool. Cut into squares. If you are going to do the chocolate drizzle, simply melt chocolate and butter together in the microwave or a double boiler. Use a spoon to drizzle chocolate over the top. You can let the drizzled bars harden at room temperature or pop them in the fridge to speed up the process.

Yields 18-20 small squares.

Gluten Free. Smart Carb.

CHOCOLATE PROTEIN ZUCCHINI BREAD

A great way to use up some extra zucchini from the garden or farmers market that will give you a moist, melt in your mouth treat, all without the extra carbs.

Ingredients

1 medium zucchini, shredded (equal to 1 1/2 cups shredded zucchini)
2 eggs, whisked
3/4 cup almond or peanut butter
1/3 cup honey
1/4 cup cocoa powder
2 Tbsp coconut flour
1 scoop of chocolate whey or plant protein
1 tsp vanilla extract
1 tsp cinnamon
1/2 tsp baking powder
1/2 tsp baking soda
Pinch of salt

Instructions

Preheat your oven to 375°F. Shred your zucchini. Use the shredding attachment on your food processor or using a cheese grater. Once your zucchini is shredded, you need to remove the excess liquid. Place a couple of paper towels or dish towel down on the counter, throw the zucchini on top, then place another paper towel on top of the zucchini then squeeze. Use more paper towels as needed, but be sure to squeeze until the zucchini feels waterless. Place zucchini in a bowl with the rest of your ingredients. Use a large spoon to mix well until all the ingredients are combined and you have a deep chocolate colour. Pour your ingredients into a greased non-stick loaf pan. Place in oven to bake for 30-35 minutes or until toothpick comes out clean when you poke it. Remove from oven and flip bread out gently onto a cooling rack. Let cool to slice and serve.

Yields one loaf.

Gluten Free. Smart Carb.

KETO PSYLLIUM HUSK BREAD

With a hearty but moist texture, this keto bread slices and serves almost as good as traditional bread but without the carbs. It is great for keto diet sandwiches or just a snack when smeared with some nut butter or avocado.

Dry Ingredients

6 Tbsp psyllium husks
1 cup coconut flour or
1 1/2 cups almond flour
1 tsp salt

Optional spices, to taste: (garlic powder, Parmesan, oregano)
1 1/2 tsp baking soda

Wet Ingredients

1/2 cup extra-virgin olive oil or avocado oil
1/4 cup coconut oil

3/4 cup warm water
8 whole eggs (or 2 cups eggs whites)

Instructions

Preheat oven to 350°F. In a large bowl mix together dry ingredients, then add wet ingredients, and mix all together. Pour your ingredients into a greased non-stick loaf pan. Place in oven to bake for 45-55 minutes or until toothpick comes out clean when you poke it. Remove from oven and flip bread out gently onto a cooling rack. Let cool to slice and serve.

Yields one loaf.

Gluten Free. Low Carb. Keto

SWEET POTATO PROTEIN BARS

No-bake protein bars with great taste and texture thanks to sweet potatoes. That's sweeeeeet!

Ingredients

1 large cooked sweet potato (peel removed)
1 scoop of vanilla whey or plant protein
1 Tbsp honey
1 Tbsp of coconut flour
1 Tbsp of ground flaxseed
2 Tbsp of unsweetened coconut milk
1/2 bar of 85% dark chocolate

Instructions

In a large bowl, mix all the ingredients (except for the chocolate) together. Shape the mixture into four little bars and put aside. Melt your chocolate either in a double boiler (a glass bowl fitted over a smaller pot of boiling water) or in a small, non-metal bowl, using low power, in the microwave. Once melted, dip your bars in the chocolate until they are fully coated. Place them on a cookie sheet lined with wax or parchment paper, or into a large plastic or freezer-safe glass container. Transfer them to the freezer for an hour, or the fridge overnight.

Yields 4 bars.

Gluten Free. Smart Carb.

FROZEN BANANA BITES

Heat up some dark chocolate and cool down some bananas, to bite into this decadent dessert.

Ingredients

2 large bananas
1/4 cup dark chocolate chips

1/4 cup natural peanut butter or almond butter
1/4 cup unsweetened coconut flakes

Instructions

Set out a large plate or bowl with a piece of parchment or wax paper on it. Cut up the bananas into good-sized chunks. Each banana should give you around 5 to 6 pieces. Heat the peanut butter and chocolate chips in the microwave on high for about a minute. Then stir until smooth.

Dip the banana pieces in the chocolate-peanut butter mixture. Lay them out, leaving some space between them on the parchment/wax paper. Then when you've covered them all, use the remaining mixture to spoon over the tops. Then sprinkle the unsweetened coconut flakes on top. Transfer to the freezer for about an hour until hardened (if you can't wait) or better to cover them with some plastic wrap or place in a flat, plastic container and let freeze overnight.

2 servings.

Gluten Free. Smart Carb.

MICROWAVED MUG CHOCOLATE CAKE

Ingredients

2 Tbsp gluten-free flour blend
1 Tbsp natural powdered sweetener (stevia or coconut sugar)
2 tsp unsweetened cocoa powder
1/4 tsp baking powder

Pinch of salt
1 tsp butter or coconut oil, melted
2 Tbsp unsweetened almond milk
1/8 tsp pure vanilla extract
3/4 Tbsp mini chocolate chips, divided

Instructions

Grab a 1/2 cup capacity mug or ramekin and spray with avocado oil or grease with coconut oil or butter. Into the mug, add in the flour, sweetener, cocoa powder, baking powder and salt. Whisk to combine. Add melted butter, milk, and vanilla. Fold in 1/2 tablespoon of chocolate chips. Mix them through. Top with the remaining chocolate chips.

Minute Microwave Method: Bake in your microwave on the quick or high setting for 40 seconds. Open the door and gently touch the top with your fingertip. If it's still a little underdone in the middle, microwave for another 10 seconds until cooked through (not too long, as the cake will continue cooking in the mug once it's removed).

Oven Baked Version: Preheat oven to 350°F. Spray a 1/2 cup capacity ramekin with cooking oil spray. Prepare as above and bake in the oven for around 15 minutes, or until a toothpick inserted into the centre comes out clean. (For a fudgier cake, check it after 11 minutes with a toothpick and it should come out slightly sticky, but not with a lot of cake batter attached.)

1 serving.

Gluten Free. Smart Carb.

20 EASY EATING KITCHEN TIPS AND TRICKS

1. **Bake your Bacon.** It is called BAKE-IN after all! For evenly browned bacon that doesn't splatter grease and curl up, line a baking sheet with parchment paper, lay out slices of bacon slightly apart, and pop in a 400°F oven for 20 minutes. Better bacon and easy eating cleanup.

2. **Egg Crack Hack.** Crack eggs on a flat surface, like your counter top, instead of a sharp edge, like a bowl or knife to avoid splitting up the shells and leaving you with some shells left floating in your eggs. Take it a step further for easier clean up and lay a piece of large paper towel down on your counter before you tap and crack, for easier cleanup and collecting shells.

3. **Better Cooked Chicken.** Chicken will cook faster and more evenly if you butterfly the breast, pound it to equal thickness, and cut it into fillets first. Otherwise, the small end of the breast can get overcooked and dry by the time the larger side is cooked. It's an extra step, but makes a huge difference taste-wise, and looks so much better when plated.

4. **Preheat your Pan.** Before adding food to your pan, wait until your pan (greased with a little oil) is adequately heated before adding food to it. This will give your food a golden sear and prevent it from sticking and cooking unevenly. Just drop the heat to medium once the pan is heated up.

5. **Don't Shy from Salt.** Such a simple thing, but under-seasoning food with a good quality salt is such a common mistake, but also easily fixed. So salt to taste as you cook and if "something's missing?" it's usually a little more salt.

6. **Make the Cut.** Sharpen. Your. Knives. Cutting and chopping food with dull knives is the worst, and also dangerous! Even a cheap knife can be sharpened, but I recommend you invest in a good set. It will save you time, money, and will prove less dangerous than cutting with a dull knife. It will also help you cry less when cutting onions, because when knives are sharp, you are actually

slicing through the onions with your knife not just pushing out the juice with a dull knife and crying over your cutting board.

7. **Get a Grip.** Speaking of cutting boards, the easiest way to keep your cutting board safe and stable is to grab a dish towel, wet it, and wring it out so it's just damp, then lay it out flat on your counter before placing the cutting board down on it. That's it. The damp dish towel acts as a good grip, preventing your board from moving around. It's one of the first safety tips I taught my kids in the kitchen (after don't touch the hot burner of course!)

8. **Move your Meat.** Allow your steak to come up to room temperature before cooking it by taking it out of the fridge 30 minutes before cooking. This will allow for more even and predictable cooking. As cooking a cold steak directly from the fridge means that once it hits the hot pan or grill, the fibres in the meat go into shock, tense up, and result in a tough steak.

9. **Perfect Potatoes.** For potato dishes that are crispy on the outside and fluffy on the inside, dunk them in ice-cold water before cooking them. When making fries, hash browns, or other potato dishes from scratch, cut or grate your potatoes and immediately put the pieces into ice-cold water. This prevents potatoes from turning pink or brown and removes some of the starch, which helps make potato dishes fluffier. Just don't forget to pat them dry to remove the excess moisture. The cold dunk soak is one of the secrets many fry guy restaurants use to get the fries golden crispy on the outside but soft on the inside.

10. **Don't let the Juice Loose.** Don't cut into your meat or chicken to check if it's done—use an instant read thermometer! They only cost a few bucks and will make sure everyone has their steak cooked to their liking and nobody gets undercooked meat. Any slice or hole you poke into meat or chicken is an escape path for the important flavourful juices to run away.

11. **Omit the Oil.** In the pasta water that is. I admit, I used to do this, thinking adding olive oil to pasta water made better pasta that wouldn't stick together. But don't add olive oil to your pasta water. This actually can prevent the sauce you add from sticking to the starchy pasta. Adding lots of salt to the pasta water instead is key to better flavour.

Also, don't rinse pasta after you've drained it. Rinsing pasta removes the natural starch from the surface of the noodles and the sauce won't stick as well.

12. **Season from the Start.** Always season your vegetables at the start when you add them to the pan. This prevents over-seasoning at the end and makes the flavour even better than if you only seasoned at the end. You really should be tasting and seasoning throughout your cooking process. Your food will taste way better and you might find you don't need to use as much of it.

13. **Rinse your Rice.** For fluffy texture and restaurant like rice, rinse your rice in a fine mesh colander before cooking. This removes the surface starch from rice grains, which can make them sticky and clumpy as they cook.

14. **A Loaf Pan is a Pain.** Unless you are baking bread, choose a large baking sheet to cook your meatloaf—not a loaf pan. (Like you will see in the meatloaf recipe in this book.) A loaf pan is a pain for removing, slicing and serving the meatloaf and it traps in all the grease and fat and makes it soggy. Make and mold a free-form meatloaf on a large baking sheet so you have more room to slice and serve, and the grease drains away and the meat can brown all around.

15. **Instant Ice Coffee.** Stop diluting your daily energy boost with standard ice cubes. Instead, freeze an ice cube tray filled with your favourite coffee blend so you can cool down your hot coffee or instantly have iced coffee without watering down the taste.

16. **De-Stem Strawberries.** Here's a "berry" easy trick to remove the stem of a "straw-berry": Insert a straw through the pointy, bottom end of the strawberry and press it straight up to push the leaves out!

17. **Coat Cups and Spoons**. Avoid the mess of measuring when baking with sticky ingredients like honey, maple syrup, nut butters and other sticky ingredients. These will slip right out of measuring cups when you grease them first! Simply spray or wipe the inside of measuring cups and spoons with non-stick cooking spray or oil before adding sticky ingredients, for easier cooking cleanup.

18. **Shake it Off to Skin Garlic.** Control the mess and speed up peeling a pile of garlic cloves by separating them, popping the cloves in a mason jar, and screwing on the lid. Give the jar a good shake and the skins should slide right off, leaving you ready to mince and mingle. You can also use the same shake it off strategy with two equal-sized bowls, one held tight inverted on top of the other.

19. **Frozen Fresh Herbs.** Freeze a fresh herb mixture in olive oil to add to your meals. If you are the kind of person who likes to add fresh herbs to meals, you can stock up on herbs, chop them up, put them in an ice cube tray, cover them in olive oil and freeze them. Next time you are cooking something, just drop a cube in for fast fresh flavour.

20. **Smoothly Sliced Two-Plate Tomatoes**. Use two plates to slice small cherry tomatoes in one smooth motion. If you are making a big salad and need to chop a whole bunch of cherry tomatoes in half, just pin them between two plates (with the bottom plate upside down, and the top plate right-side up). Press down on the top plate with one hand to keep everything in place, and carefully slice through them horizontally with a sharp knife. You can slice a dozen or more of them in one clean cut!

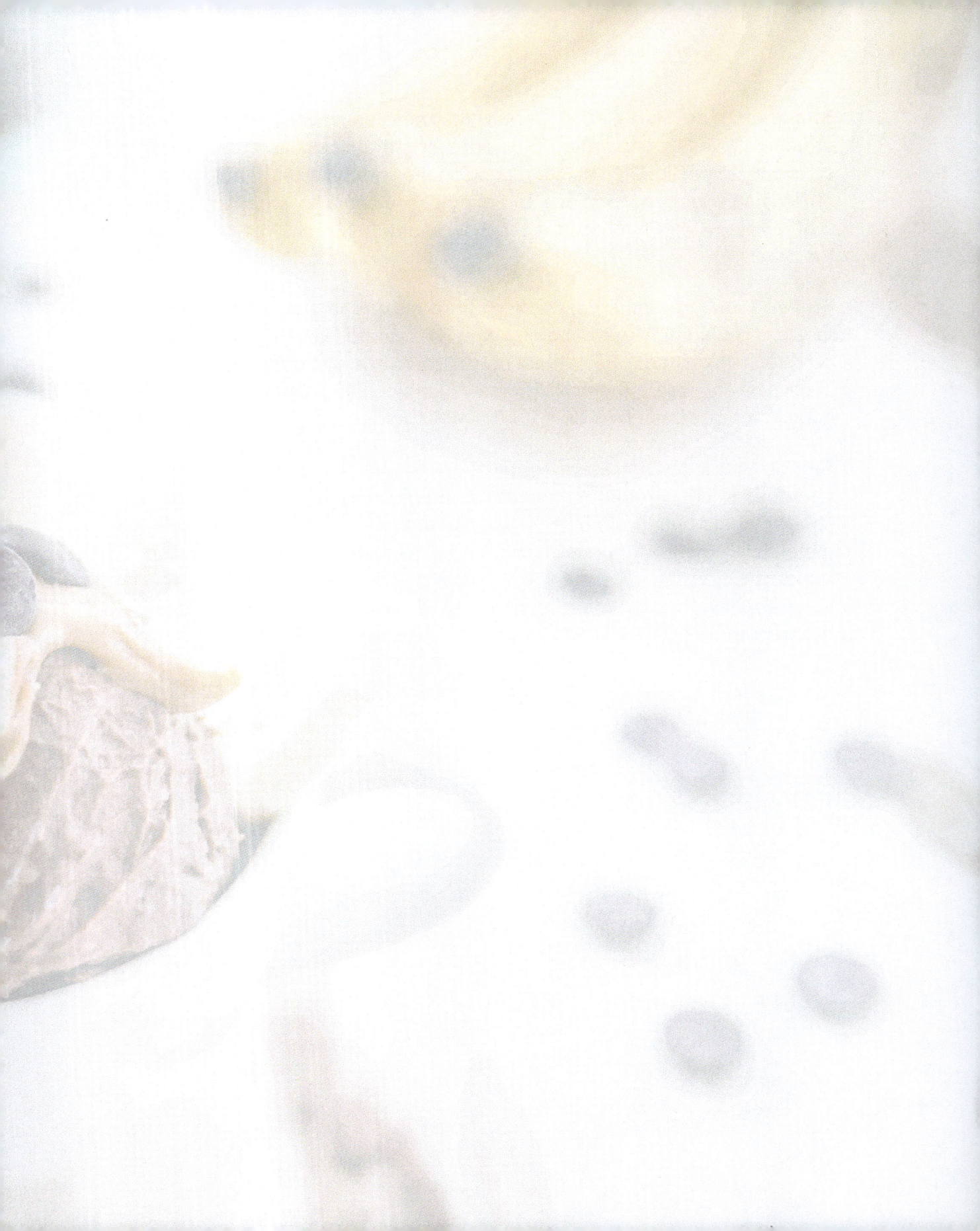

50 EASY EATING *SUPER SMOOTHIES*

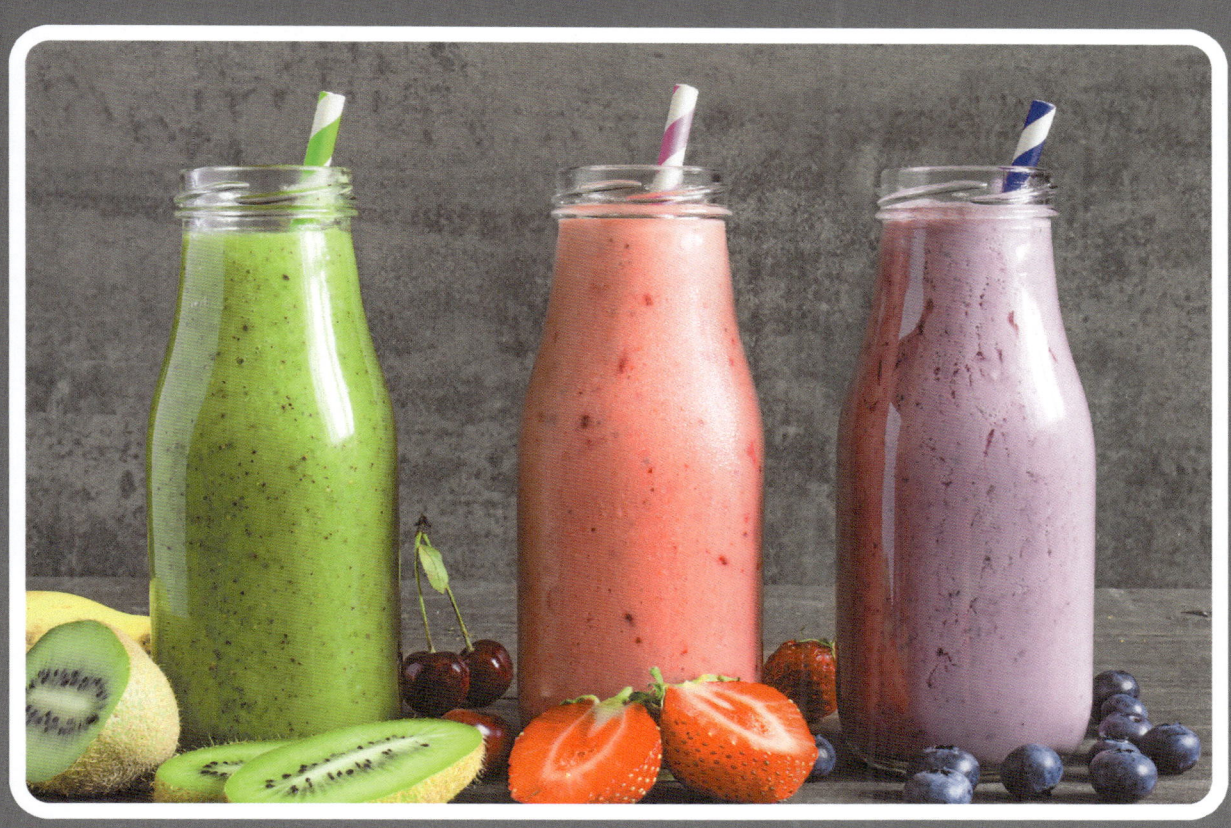

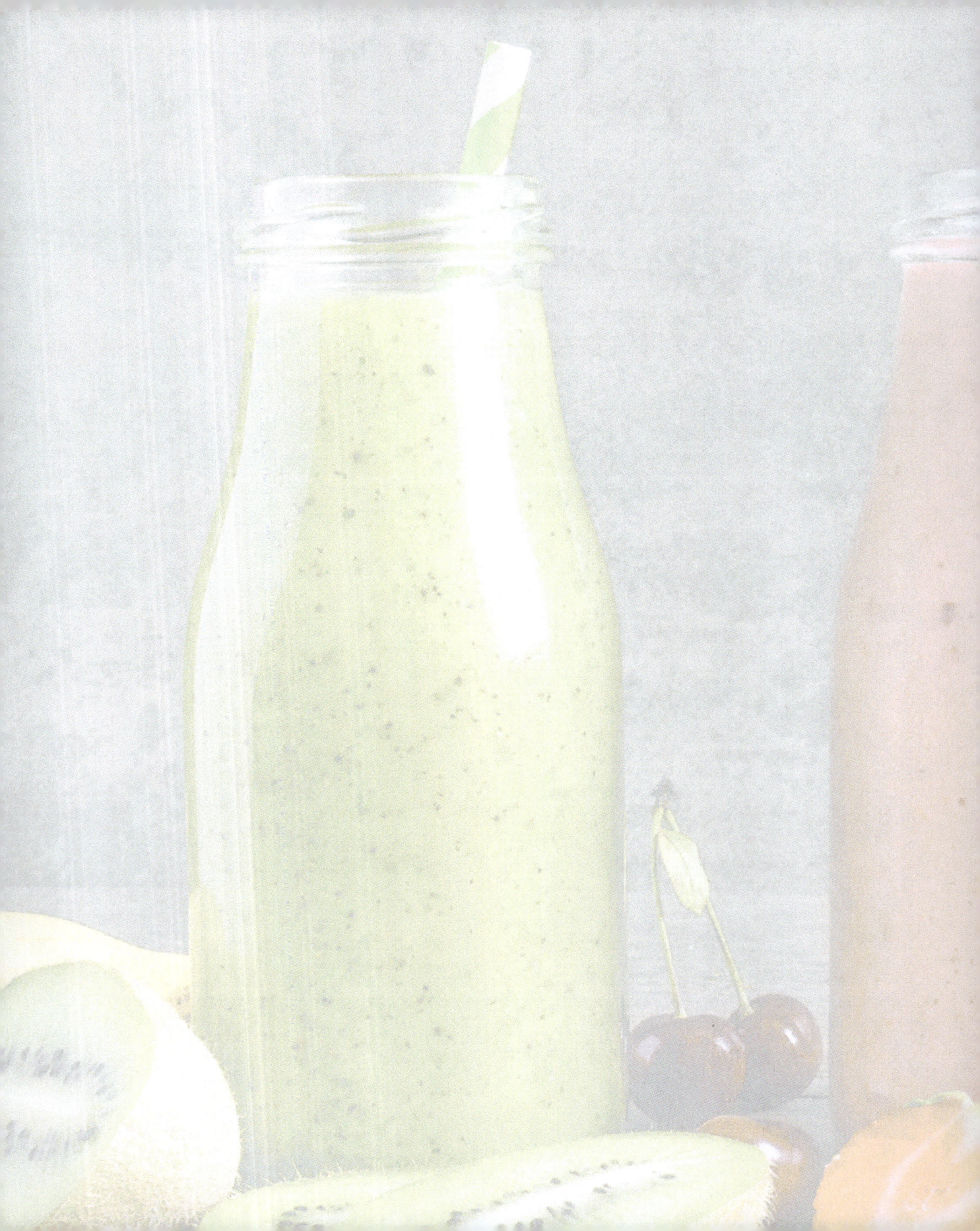

EASY EATING SUPER SMOOTHIES

Sometimes you need a quick, energy-rich breakfast before rushing out the door to go to work, or you want a light lunch you can have on your way back from the gym or in between meetings. Something that satisfies you that you can have in your car while chauffeuring around the kids (that doesn't require going through a drive-thru) or even sitting down to a table with forks and knives.

But you also want something healthy that makes you feel good and avoids a mid-morning or mid-afternoon carb coma. Something full of natural nutrients found in fruits and vegetables, high quality protein, and healthy fats. And something quick and easy. Enter the **Easy Eating Super Smoothie.** It's a minute meal in a glass, packed with high-quality liquid nutrition that gives you everything you need in a convenient, portable, delicious drink.

Meal replacement shakes are convenient for busy lifestyles, are helpful for people who struggle to eat enough nutrients (especially protein and produce), and for those controlling calories. They have been long used and proven in research and real life as an effective option to control your diet and body composition, whether for weight loss, weight maintenance, or intentional lean weight gain.

These Super Smoothies are simply delicious liquid meals that save you time, nourish your body, and satisfy you, one sip at a time. For any of the super smoothie recipes with dense, whole food ingredients, I recommend investing in a good, high-powered blender, and let it whirl for easy drinking!

For most light, liquid-based smoothies, lower-powered blenders will do the job. Along with my high-powered blender that I invested in over ten years ago (despite its daily use) it still spins strong today! But I also use one of those popular small blenders for quick, single-serving smoothies. Depending on your goals you can use a Super Smoothie as a meal replacement in place of a whole food meal (for maximum fat loss) or added in between meals (for maximum muscle gain). **Happy blending!**

Apple Cinnamon Smoothie

Ingredients

1 scoop of vanilla whey or plant protein powder
1 cup of unsweetened vanilla almond milk
1 Granny Smith apple (cored, sliced)
1/2 frozen banana
1 tsp cinnamon
Stevia sweetener, to taste
3 ice cubes

Apricot Vanilla Smoothie

Ingredients

1 scoop of vanilla whey or plant protein powder
1 cup unsweetened vanilla almond milk
1/2 cup plain Greek 2% yogurt
3 dried apricot halves
1 Tbsp honey
3 ice cubes

Banana Bread Smoothie

Ingredients

1 scoop of vanilla whey or plant protein powder
1 cup unsweetened vanilla almond milk
1/2 frozen banana
1/2 cup (dry measure) rolled oats
1 tsp cinnamon
3 ice cubes

Banana Nutella Smoothie

Ingredients

1 scoop of vanilla whey or plant protein powder
1 cup unsweetened almond milk
1/2 cup plain Greek 2% yogurt
1 Tbsp chocolate hazelnut spread
1/2 frozen banana
1/2 tsp pure vanilla extract
Stevia, to taste
3 ice cubes

Banana Split Smoothie

Ingredients

1 scoop of vanilla whey or plant protein powder
1 cup unsweetened vanilla almond milk
1/2 frozen banana
1/2 cup frozen pineapple chunks
3 frozen sliced strawberries
1 tsp pure cocoa powder
3 ice cubes

Blue Bomber Smoothie

Ingredients

1 scoop of vanilla whey or plant protein powder
1/2 cup plain Greek 2% yogurt
1 cup water
1 cup frozen blueberries
Stevia, to taste
3 ice cubes

Blueberry Bliss Smoothie

Ingredients

1 scoop of vanilla whey or plant protein powder
1 cup unsweetened almond milk
1 cup frozen blueberries
1/2 frozen banana
2 Tbsp flaxseed meal
Stevia, to taste
3 ice cubes

Carrot Cake Protein Smoothie

Ingredients

1 scoop of vanilla whey or plant protein powder
1 cup unsweetened vanilla almond milk
1/2 frozen banana
1/2 cup baby carrots
2 Tbsp flaxseed meal
1/2 tsp vanilla extract
1/2 tsp each of cinnamon and nutmeg
Stevia, to taste
3 ice cubes

Chocolate Cherry Smoothie

Ingredients

1 scoop of chocolate whey or plant protein powder
1 cup unsweetened chocolate almond milk
1/2 cup plain Greek 2% yogurt
1 cup frozen cherries
1 Tbsp honey
3 ice cubes

Creamy Peach Smoothie

Ingredients

    1 scoop of vanilla whey or plant protein powder
    1/2 cup plain Greek 2% yogurt
    1 cup water
    1 peach, pitted and sliced
    1 Tbsp honey
    3 ice cubes

Honey Raspberry Smoothie

Ingredients

    1 scoop of vanilla whey or plant protein powder
    1/2 cup plain Greek 2% yogurt
    1 cup water
    1 cup frozen raspberries
    1/2 frozen banana
    1 Tbsp honey
    3 ice cubes

Mixed Berry Smoothie

Ingredients

    1 scoop of vanilla whey or plant protein powder
    1 cup unsweetened almond milk
    1/2 cup plain Greek 2% yogurt
    1/4 cup frozen sliced strawberries
    1/4 cup frozen blueberries
    1/4 cup frozen raspberries
    1 Tbsp honey
    3 ice cubes

Oats and Honey Smoothie

Ingredients

1 scoop of vanilla whey or plant protein powder
1 cup unsweetened vanilla almond milk
1/2 cup (dry measure) rolled oats
1 Tbsp honey
Stevia, to taste
3 ice cubes

Piña Colada Smoothie

Ingredients

1 scoop of vanilla whey or plant protein powder
1 cup unsweetened vanilla almond milk
1/2 cup frozen pineapple chunks
3 Tbsp unsweetened shredded coconut
Stevia, to taste
3 ice cubes

Strawberry Banana Smoothie

Ingredients

1 scoop of vanilla whey or plant protein powder
1 cup unsweetened vanilla almond milk
1/2 frozen banana
1 cup frozen sliced strawberries
Stevia, to taste
3 ice cubes

Blueberry Banana Nut Smoothie

Ingredients

1 scoop of vanilla whey or plant protein powder
1 cup unsweetened vanilla almond milk
1/2 cup plain Greek 2% yogurt
1/2 frozen banana
1/2 cup blueberries
1 Tbsp crunchy natural peanut butter
1/2 tsp cinnamon
3 ice cubes

Tropical Smoothie

Ingredients

1 scoop of vanilla whey or plant protein powder
1 cup unsweetened coconut milk
1/2 cup honeydew melon
1/2 frozen banana
1/2 cup mango
3 Tbsp unsweetened shredded coconut
Stevia, to taste
3 ice cubes

Banana Coconut Smoothie

Ingredients

1 scoop of vanilla whey or plant protein powder
1 cup unsweetened coconut milk
3 Tbsp unsweetened shredded coconut
1/2 frozen banana
1 tsp coconut extract
3 ice cubes

Berries and Cream Smoothie

Ingredients

1 scoop of vanilla whey or plant protein powder
1 cup unsweetened almond milk
1/2 cup 2% cottage cheese
1/2 cup frozen sliced strawberries
1/2 cup frozen blueberries
2 Tbsp flaxseed meal
3 ice cubes

Chocolate Covered Strawberry Smoothie

Ingredients

1 scoop chocolate whey or plant protein powder
1 cup unsweetened chocolate almond milk
1 cup frozen sliced strawberries
2 Tbsp flaxseed meal
Stevia, to taste
3 ice cubes

Chocolate Lover's Smoothie

Ingredients

1 scoop chocolate whey or plant protein powder
1 cup unsweetened chocolate almond milk
1 Tbsp pure cocoa powder
1 Tbsp natural peanut butter
1/2 frozen banana
1/2 Tbsp extra-virgin coconut oil
Stevia, to taste
3 ice cubes

Chocolate Orange Smoothie

Ingredients

1 scoop chocolate whey or plant protein powder
1 cup unsweetened chocolate almond milk
1/2 cup low-fat cottage cheese
1 orange, peeled, segmented, and all skin removed
2 Tbsp flaxseed meal
Stevia, to taste
3 ice cubes

Cinnamon Roll Supreme Smoothie

Ingredients

1 scoop of vanilla whey or plant protein powder
1 cup unsweetened vanilla almond milk
1 tsp cinnamon
1/2 tsp vanilla extract
1 tsp butter extract
Stevia, to taste
3 ice cubes

Green Superfood Smoothie

Ingredients

1 scoop of vanilla whey or plant protein powder
1 cup water
1 cup baby spinach or kale leaves, ribs and stems removed 1/2 frozen banana
3 Tbsp unsweetened coconut flakes
Stevia, to taste
3 ice cubes

Green Tea Protein Smoothie

Ingredients

1 scoop of vanilla whey or plant protein powder
1 cup unsweetened vanilla almond milk
1/2 frozen banana
1 Tbsp of greens powder or matcha green tea
Stevia, to taste
3 ice cubes

Peanut Butterscotch Smoothie

Ingredients

1 scoop of vanilla whey or plant protein powder
1 cup unsweetened vanilla almond milk
1/2 cup plain 2% Greek yogurt
1 tsp butter extract
1 Tbsp natural peanut butter
Stevia, to taste
3 ice cubes

Peanut Butter and Banana Delight Smoothie

Ingredients

1 scoop of vanilla whey or plant protein powder
1 cup unsweetened almond milk
1/2 cup low-fat cottage cheese
1/2 frozen banana
1 Tbsp natural peanut butter
Stevia, to taste
3 ice cubes

Peanut Butter Cup Smoothie

Ingredients

1 scoop chocolate whey or plant protein powder
1 cup unsweetened chocolate almond milk
1/2 frozen banana
2 Tbsp natural peanut butter
1 Tbsp pure cocoa powder
Stevia, to taste
3 ice cubes

Popeye's Super Spinach Smoothie

Ingredients

1 scoop of vanilla whey or plant protein powder
1 cup unsweetened almond milk
2 cups baby spinach
1/2 frozen banana
1 Tbsp of extra-virgin "olive oil"
Stevia, to taste
3 ice cubes

Strawberry Cheesecake Smoothie

Ingredients

1 scoop of vanilla whey or plant protein powder
1 cup unsweetened vanilla almond milk
1/2 cup plain 2% Greek yogurt
1 cup frozen sliced strawberries
1/2 tsp cinnamon
Stevia, to taste
3 ice cubes

Strawberry Shortcake Smoothie

Ingredients

1 scoop of vanilla whey or plant protein powder
1 cup unsweetened vanilla almond milk
5 frozen sliced strawberries
1/2 tsp almond extract
Stevia, to taste
3 ice cubes

Veggie Lover's Smoothie

Ingredients

1 scoop of vanilla whey or plant protein powder
1 cup unsweetened vanilla almond milk
1/2 cup plain 2% Greek yogurt
1 cup baby spinach
1/4 cup each: baby carrots, avocado, cucumber
1/2 Tbsp coconut oil
1 Tbsp cashews
3 ice cubes

Café Mocha Smoothie

Ingredients

1 scoop chocolate whey or plant protein powder
1/4 cup unsweetened vanilla almond milk
1/2 cup cold brewed coffee
2 Tbsp flaxseed meal
Stevia, to taste
3 ice cubes

Cake Batter Smoothie

Ingredients

1 scoop of vanilla whey or plant protein powder
1 cup unsweetened vanilla almond milk
1/2 cup low-fat cottage cheese
1/2 tsp pure vanilla extract
Stevia, to taste
3 ice cubes

Chocolate Coconut Smoothie

Ingredients

1 scoop chocolate whey or plant protein powder
1 cup unsweetened chocolate almond milk
1 Tbsp natural almond butter
3 Tbsp unsweetened shredded coconut
Stevia, to taste
3 ice cubes

Chocolate Covered Almond Joy Smoothie

Ingredients

1 scoop chocolate whey or plant protein powder
1 cup unsweetened coconut milk
1 Tbsp shredded coconut
1/2 oz almonds
1/2 tsp almond extract
1 Tbsp pure cocoa powder
Stevia, to taste
3 ice cubes

Chocolate Turtle Smoothie

Ingredients

1 scoop chocolate whey or plant protein powder
1 cup unsweetened chocolate almond milk
1/3 cup liquid egg whites (pasteurized)
2 Tbsp flaxseed meal
1 Tbsp almond butter or 1/4 cup chopped pecans
Stevia, to taste
3 ice cubes

Choco-Mint Smoothie

Ingredients

1 scoop chocolate whey or plant protein powder
1 cup unsweetened chocolate almond milk
1 tsp pure cocoa powder
2 tsp mint extract
Stevia, to taste
3 ice cubes

Coconut Protein Smoothie

Ingredients

1 scoop of vanilla whey or plant protein powder
1 cup unsweetened almond milk
1 Tbsp extra-virgin coconut oil
1/2 frozen banana
Stevia, to taste
3 ice cubes

Creamy Vanilla Mint Smoothie

Ingredients

    1 scoop of vanilla whey or plant protein powder
    1 cup unsweetened vanilla almond milk
    3 Tbsp heavy whipping cream
    3-6 drops mint extract
    Stevia, to taste
    3 ice cubes

Cup o' Joe Smoothie

Ingredients

    1 scoop of vanilla whey or plant protein powder
    1 cup cold brewed coffee
    1 cup unsweetened chocolate almond milk
    1/2 frozen banana
    Stevia, to taste
    3 ice cubes

Lean Leprechaun Smoothie

Ingredients

    1 scoop of vanilla whey or plant protein powder
    1 cup unsweetened almond milk
    1/2 cup low-fat cottage cheese
    1/2 tsp mint extract
    1 serving of greens powder
    Stevia, to taste
    3 ice cubes

Mochaccino Smoothie

Ingredients

1 scoop chocolate whey or plant protein powder
1 cup cold brewed coffee
1/2 cup unsweetened chocolate almond milk
1 Tbsp pure cocoa powder
Stevia, to taste
3 ice cubes

Nuts & Flax Smoothie

Ingredients

1 scoop of vanilla whey or plant protein powder
1 cup unsweetened almond milk
1/2 cup low-fat cottage cheese
2 Tbsp flaxseed meal
1/2 oz walnuts
1/2 oz almonds
Stevia, to taste
3 ice cubes

Orange Creamsicle Smoothie

Ingredients

1 scoop of vanilla whey or plant protein powder
1 cup unsweetened vanilla almond milk
1 Tbsp heavy whipping cream
1 tsp pure orange extract or 1/2 peeled segmented orange
2 Tbsp flaxseed meal
Stevia, to taste
3 ice cubes

PB & J Protein Smoothie

Ingredients

1 scoop of vanilla whey or plant protein powder
1 cup unsweetened almond milk
1/2 cup low-fat cottage cheese
1 Tbsp natural peanut butter
5 frozen sliced strawberries
Stevia, to taste
3 ice cubes

Pumpkin Pie Smoothie

Ingredients

1 scoop of vanilla whey or plant protein powder
1 cup unsweetened almond milk
1/2 cup canned pumpkin puree
1 tsp cinnamon
1/2 tsp nutmeg
Stevia, to taste
3 ice cubes

Strawberry Macadamia Nut Smoothie

Ingredients

1 scoop of vanilla whey or plant protein powder
1 cup unsweetened vanilla almond milk
1/2 cup frozen sliced strawberries
1 oz macadamia nuts
Stevia, to taste
3 ice cubes

Vanilla Almond Swirl Smoothie

Ingredients

1 scoop of vanilla whey or plant protein powder
1 cup unsweetened vanilla almond milk
1 Tbsp almond butter
1/2 tsp almond extract
1/2 tsp pumpkin pie spice
Stevia, to taste
3 ice cubes

Vanilla and Flax Smoothie

Ingredients

1 scoop of vanilla whey or plant protein powder
1 cup unsweetened vanilla almond milk
1/2 cup plain 2% Greek yogurt
2 Tbsp flaxseed meal
1 tsp pure vanilla extract
Stevia, to taste
3 ice cubes

THANK YOU

We hope this cookbook has inspired you, given you confidence and clarity in the kitchen, and has provided you with lifelong skills to be healthier and happier.

Rise up and reach out to join our movement at Easy Eating. We would love to hear from you, whether it's about the book, press or media interviews, speaking, writing, podcasts, book signings, general inquiries, collaboration, or opportunities. And be sure to tag us on social media with what you have cooking in *your* kitchen!

To contact us and stay up-to-date on all things regarding *The Easy Eating Diet* and The *Easy Eating Diet Cookbook* please visit us on the web at **www.EasyEatingDiet.com** and at The Easy Eating Diet on Facebook and on Instagram @sbarker78.

It would be greatly appreciated if after reading *The Easy Eating Diet* or *The Easy Eating Diet Cookbook*, you take a minute to leave a review on Amazon.

From my home to yours. Thank You!

Printed in Great Britain
by Amazon